RAVENS AND RAINBOWS

A Mother-Daughter Story of Grit, Courage, and Love After Death

L. Grey
Vanessa Lynn, Ph.D.

Copyright © 2020 Defining Moments Press, Inc and Vanessa Lynn

All rights reserved. No part of this book may be reproduced in any form without permission in writing from the author. Reviewers may quote brief passages in reviews.

DISCLAIMER No part of this publication may be reproduced or transmitted in any form or by any means, mechanical or electronic, including

photocopying or recording, or by any information storage and retrieval system, or transmitted by email without permission in writing from the

author. Neither the author nor the publisher assumes any responsibility for

errors, omissions, or contrary interpretations of the subject matter herein.

Any perceived slight of any individual or organization is purely unintentional. Brand and product names are trademarks or registered trademarks of their respective owners.

Although the author and publisher have made every effort to ensure that the information in this book was correct at press time, the author and publisher do not assume and hereby disclaim any liability to any party for any loss,

damage, or disruption caused by errors or omissions, whether such errors or omissions result from negligence, accident, or any other cause.

This book is not intended as a substitute for the medical advice of physicians.

The reader should regularly consult a physician in matters relating to his/her health and particularly with respect to any symptoms that may require diagnosis or medical attention.

Editing: Amber Cherie Torres, Linda Sweeney and Jennifer Rosenthal

RAVENS
AND
RAINBOWS

A Mother-Daughter Story of Grit, Courage, and Love After Death

L. Grey

Vanessa Lynn, Ph.D.

"Candidly, this book broke me and put me back together in a way that goes beyond emotion. This literature is alive. The experience of reading it connects you not only to L, but to the world and to your own soul, naturally pushing you to be more introspective."
–H. Miller

I am blessed to have known L as a student. I would need her gift with words to more eloquently describe her impact on me, our school, and all those she met. There's strong, and then there is L Strong. Wit, and then L Wit. Tenacity, and then L Tenacity. There are so many categories where L is a simply like no other. This story will take you to places of heartbreak, laughter, and the unrelenting love between a mother and a daughter.
–T. Costello

There is nothing like this book that L and Vanessa have meticulously created. It's a gift to all of us. Borrow their bravery, build some of your own, and better the world.
–A. Wernick

*For L
You made it… with all the truth in the world
I love you more than anything
-Momma*

TABLE OF CONTENTS

PROLOGUE

In April 2015, life was relatively uncomplicated. I was 41 years old and living in suburban Chicago with my two daughters. L. Grey was 12, a precocious girl with wisdom beyond her years, curiosity beyond measure, and a sixth sense beyond anyone's comprehension. She was an enigma, who was intensely private and yet also determined to be a loud voice in the world. At an early age, she shortened her given name to the letter L, and later adopted the pseudonym Grey so she could write, blog, and podcast fearlessly while still maintaining her privacy. Jaz was 10, the picture of childhood innocence, whose hugs could melt away any problem and whose world revolved around her friends, hip-hop dance, and baking cupcakes.

I wrestled with the things that most professionals my age likely wrestled with: balancing the demands of an exacting career as a consultant with the gravitational pull to be with my girls as often as I could, trying to figure out how to be a good mom while simultaneously being the family breadwinner. All in all, we had a pretty good rhythm. I traveled often for work, but I'd do whatever I could to be home at night, so 5:00 am flights were a regular part of my week, and somehow I had managed to be the "room mom" for every Halloween and Valentine's Day party at school; I had never missed a recital or school event. In the grand scheme of things, our world was as close to being balanced as it could be, and our future was full of hope and promise.

On April 21, 2015, L twisted her ankle at school. What should have been a non-event ended up crippling L with a debilitating disease that ravaged her body in ways we never could have imagined, and it ultimately cost her her life. She was diagnosed with Complex Regional Pain Syndrome (CRPS), a neurological condition that causes the brain to send pain signals to parts of the body, causing unrelenting pain and creating the sensation of being burned alive.

Over the course of her three-and-a-half-year illness, she became confined to a wheelchair, then to her bed. She would be in constant burning pain, and her major organ systems would shut down. She would reveal secrets that no parent ever wants to face. Our family would be tested, shattered, and reformulated. She would fiercely protect her sister, even from within the four walls of her room. She would build enduring friendships with people she never got to meet in person. She would become an outspoken advocate for social justice. She would show strength and courage that, to this day, I can't fully understand. She would fight until her last moment, and in the end she would teach us all about the unwavering strength of her spirit.

When she came home from school on that Spring day, there is no way I could have predicted what would follow; there is no way I could have known what was in store. But L knew. She was prescient. She knew it all, from her first breath to her last.

Introduction

On July 22, 2018, my daughter L Grey quietly filled a bath with warm water, slipped into the tub holding her beloved stuffed cow Grazer, swallowed a bottle of Norco, and closed her eyes for the last time. We would say she took her life. In the months since her passing, I have come to believe that she took her life *back*. She was 15. This is her story. This is her truth.

PART I: Before

July 2002

I was five-months pregnant with L, and we were in Sanibel Island, Florida, with my sister, my dad, and his wife. Although I grew up in suburban Chicago, Sanibel is home for me. It is where I spent my childhood vacations, and it is where L and her younger sister Jaz would spend theirs. While there, my sister penned this poem in anticipation of her birth.

Untitled
Auntie "D"
July 2002

You, who have not yet arrived at your name,
What shall I call you?
Our unopened future,
A gibbous moon, a question mark,
There is no silence like yours.
Mute coalescence in a floating world,
Darkness of water, sentience of wave; A
mollusk, a ribbon, a thumbprint, a bee.
There is no blindness like yours,
Days slowly rocking from midnight to noon,
The fiction of time measured by light;
A garnet, a raindrop, an olive, a knot.

There is no patience like yours,
Involute one, reticent as winter,
You're weaving your secret history;
A spool, a spoonful, a knuckle, a star.
There is no persistence like yours,
While we hold our breath,
Turning, turning in a liquid hush,
Hope into muscle, wish into
flesh, Tiny red heart beating;
I will. I will.

Like many expectant parents, I wanted her in-utero experience to be a positive one, so I was constantly playing music to her—anything from my favorite rock tunes to timeless classical pieces. I had never thought of music as having a defining role in her story, or in my story, or in our story. I had always enjoyed music and was thrilled when I stumbled across a song with a good running beat, but I had never really paid attention to song titles or lyrics. After L's death, I realized that music had always been an integral part of her story and our journey together, and that it would continue to be inextricably woven into our next chapter, with L gone from her body but alive and strong in spirit. When I was pregnant, I'd often listen to Phish's "Free," not thinking much of the words:

I'm floating in the blimp a lot
I feel the feeling I forgot
Swimming weightless in the womb
Bouncing gently round the room
In a minute I'll be free and we'll be splashing in the sea
I feel no curiosity
I see the path ahead of me
In a minute I'll be free
And we'll be splashing in the sea
We hear a tiny cry As
the ship goes sliding by Free!
Free!

Ironically, one of my other favorite songs to play for her while I was pregnant was Sarah Brightman and Andrea Bocelli's rendition of "Time to say Goodbye." After she was born, I turned this song into our own lullaby, making up words to the melody.

Time to go to sleep, my sweet baby girl, it is now time to close your eyes and go to sleep.

I'll be right here in the morning, when you wake up, but now it is time to go to sleep, I love you, my sweet baby girl.

November 12, 2002 2:52 am

When L was born, the delivery could only be described as exhilarating. A couple pushes, and there she was. I can remember the nurse seeing the crown of her head, realizing she was really about to come into this world and cheering me to push with all my might. The nurses plopped this warm, beautiful angel on my chest, and my life changed forever. The practical, rather unemotive woman I had been instantly disappeared as I was transformed into a mother who felt L's every emotion and was guided not by practicality or pragmatism, but by intuition and instinct.

In the background, Aerosmith's "Dream On" was playing.

Sing with me
Sing for the year
Sing for the laughter, and sing for the tear
Sing with me if it's just for today, maybe tomorrow the good lord will take you away...

"Dream On" became our family song for L. It was her anthem of sorts, and I would crank up the radio every time it came on, remembering the magic of the night of her birth. It was only after her death that I paused to actually listen to the haunting words.

October 29, 2003 (age 11 months)

It was a perfect fall day, cool and crisp, the leaves painting a rainbow on the trees. L was at that irritable age of trying to go from three naps a day down to two, and late afternoons were tough. She wasn't tired enough to fall asleep on her own in her crib, but she was cranky and out of sorts and too tired to play. I wanted to take her for a walk, but the stroller sometimes made her fussy, and in truth, I wanted to feel her on my skin. I assembled the Baby Björn, even though I knew she was really too big for it. I put it on the largest setting and squeezed her in.

At almost a year old, it was kind of comical, squishing her into this contraption, but she was snug and content, and we set off on our way. She fell asleep quickly, her eyes gently closing as her head became heavy against my chest. I knew this was borrowed time, that she was getting older and that I would have precious few moments for her to sleep on my chest, so I decided to walk for as long as she was asleep, to take in every second that she granted me.

We spent three hours walking that afternoon, just the two of us, with the fall air cool and brisk against my face, leaves crunching under-foot, the scent of L's hair filling my breath, and the sublime weight of her head against my chest, her rhythmic breathing warm against my neck. One of the many gifts L would give me was the quiet knowing that we were doing things that we would likely not be able to do again, so that I never took them for granted. So that I could savor every moment.

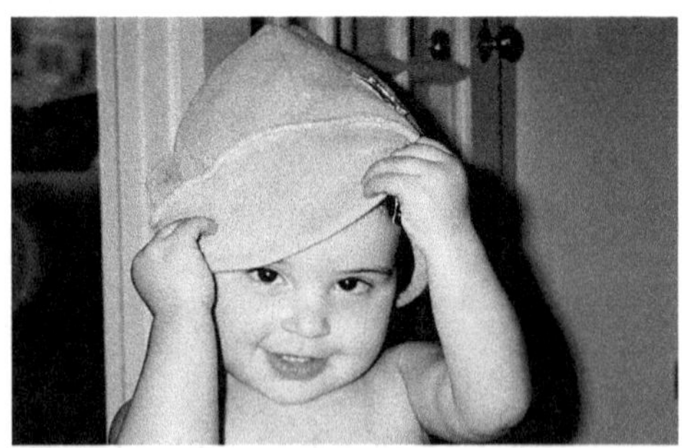

L at 11 months.

The early years, 2003–2008 (ages 1–5)

It was clear from very early on that L was not a typical child. As I look back, I can now see that she was never fully of this world. She was prescient, she knew *everything.* She sensed things that no one could quite explain. Of course, all children are unique, but there was something about L. She was exceptionally bright, but so are many children. This was different. As a baby it was clear that she understood things, felt things that were beyond her years and beyond what she could surmise from her physical surroundings. At six months old, she understood dark humor, lit up when sarcasm entered a conversation, and shrieked with laughter when I would make up games and stories with subtle plot lines, edgy characters, and sophisticated punchlines.

She discovered SpongeBob at 12 months old. We were at the grocery store. She was sitting in the front of the cart and, as we were wheeling down the cookie aisle, she spotted a box of animal crackers that had the image of SpongeBob and his sidekick Patrick on it. She pointed and started laughing hysterically. She didn't know their names. She just referred to them as yellow square and pink guy, but just looking at them made her squeal with delight. I quickly went out and bought a VHS tape of SpongeBob episodes, and L was hooked.

At 12 months old, subtle lines, like SpongeBob asking Patrick, "How stupid are you?" and Patrick replying, "It varies," or SpongeBob exclaiming, "Patrick, your genius is showing!" and Patrick blushing, covering his crotch with his hands, and asking, "It is? Where?" would have L howling with devious laughter. SpongeBob became a favorite for years to come. We could quote entire episodes. As L got older, she began to realize how much sexual innuendo was embedded in each episode, and her affinity for the show grew even more.

She became quite proud of her younger self. She was pleased with the wisdom and foresight she'd had to like a show that was so off-color. She loved the double entendres. It was her kind of humor.

When she became sick, she would occasionally let Jaz and me watch some SpongeBob episodes with her. Despite her pain, genuine delight would shine through as she applauded the sneakiness of the writers and was transported to a simpler time. "I'm really feeling it now, Mr. Krabs," became a phrase she would use on a daily basis.

L was two and a half the first time she saw fireworks on the Fourth of July. She was typically in bed by 7:00, but I thought she was old enough to stay up late and see her first fireworks show. I'll admit I was nervous. L was not the kind of kid who easily rolled with the punches, and when her sleep cycle was off, it was not a pretty sight. And her senses were so finely tuned that things like bright lights, loud noises, and big crowds tended to overwhelm her, and she would quickly look for respite. Nevertheless, I figured the worst that could happen was she would hate the fireworks and I would need to quickly whisk her home. Jaz was only a year old at the time, too little to go, so she stayed home while I took L.

We spread out our blanket and ate popcorn while we waited for it to get dark enough for the show to start. The music started and the sky began to light up. I was prepared to place my hands over her ears if the noise was too loud, but as soon as the show began, my fears were put to rest. A smile crept across her face, and she stood up as if she were lifted by an imaginary rope. She reached out, opening and closing her chubby, two-year-old hand, trying to catch each firework as it exploded in the air. She stayed like that for the whole show, grinning from ear to ear, completely unfazed by, and seemingly unaware of, the crowds around her. When the show ended, she smiled up at me and simply said, "More."

As a little girl L was slow to trust—very slow to trust. "Stranger danger" took on a whole new meaning for her. She did not show much interest in other children one way or another (although a day at the park with no one else there was delightful for her), but she would make it very clear how she felt about adults. If she trusted you, she would engage for hours. If she didn't, you could not come near her. It was that simple. If she did not trust "the adult in charge," there was no approaching her. It was not just a child having a tantrum. In fact, there was never a tantrum quality to her tears; rather, if L was crying, it was clear that it was because she was profoundly uncomfortable with a person or a situation. And if she was happy, it was clear it was because she trusted the person she was with.

As a baby, if someone looking at her gave her a bad vibe, she would immediately start crying. People would constantly offer their unsolicited perspectives: I was too protective. I should let her cry it out. I should leave her in the care of people who were not immediate family so she could "learn" to be with others and "get over" her stranger danger. I was stifling her socially. *But I knew my child.* I knew that, even though she was a baby, there was something bigger going on, something others expected her to shake off, but something I was not willing to. I worked hard to make L's world safe for her, despite ridicule from some people. When she became verbal at age two and was able to put words to her feelings, it became more clear what was going on.

We sat playing on the living room floor, surrounded by toys, when she started describing her great grandmother in specific detail. Not just the way she looked, but her personality, her humor, how she dressed, and expressions she would use. Perhaps this would not be so unusual had her great grandmother been living, but she had been gone for over 20 years, and while she was beloved, she did not ever come up in conversations, and L had never seen a picture of her.

"How do you know so much about your great grandma?" I asked.

"Well, duh, she comes in my room and hangs out with me every night." She then took a big swig of apple juice from her sippy cup, tossing her head back as she did, "Damn good juice, damn good."

Soon after that she told me about the spirit who visited her, whom L had named Penny because of the pennies over her eyes. A quick Google search taught me that the tradition of placing coins over the eyes of the deceased dates back hundreds, if not thousands, of years. L was a smart kid, but at age two, even with all her brilliance, she had not known how to do a Google search. There is no way she should have known that.

I learned that L's extrasensory abilities applied to the living as well. She just *knew* if someone was trustworthy or not. At age four, while we were having lunch at our favorite hotdog stand, a man I knew walked by. He was not a nice man, not a man whose company I would seek; in fact, he was known in the community as a pretty shady character. He and I did the polite thing and gave each other the quiet head nod, acknowledging that we saw each other but making no effort to engage in conversation.

"Do you know him?" L asked.

"Yes, I know him."

"Never mind, then. If you're friends with him, I won't say anything."

"L," I said, "I didn't say I was friends with him; I just said I knew him. What do you want to tell me?"

"He's a bad guy. Stay away from him. That's all. Can I have more fries?"

One of the things I marveled at as a young parent was how quickly, distinctly, and completely the unique personalities of the girls took shape. L's sarcasm, edginess, and insistence on marching to the beat of her own drum were matched with Jaz's innocence, sweetness, and complete adoration for her sister. It was a fascinating dynamic—L longing for independence and Jaz determined to stay as close as possible. Yet, as different as they were, they shared an incredible empathy for people, and they gave grace to one another that neither would give to anyone else.

On the surface, L would be annoyed by her little sister crowding her space, but she never fought it all that hard; her protective instinct seeming to override any mild (or perhaps not so mild) annoyance she may have been feeling. So, when Jaz started preschool at age three and was feeling homesick, L didn't flinch when Jaz left her classroom of three-year-old's and toddled into L's classroom of four- and five-year-old's where Jaz made herself quite comfortable shadowing her sister's every move for the rest of the school year.

When Jaz threw up on L's treasured blanket on an airplane, L didn't shed a tear; she just rubbed Jaz's head. L didn't argue when Jaz would wait to see what L was going to wear in the morning before dressing her-self in the identical outfit. She allowed Jaz to call her nicknames that the rest of us were forbidden to even speak, like Elly-Belly and Mo (a charac-ter from *The Doodlebops*—don't ask!). In return, Jaz would indulge L by playing whatever game L wanted (including "apartment," which would involve long stretches of each girl being alone in their own "apartments").

She would laugh when L named her Plumhead in the bathtub (to be fair, the smoothness of Jaz's wet hair bore remarkable resemblance to a plum). She thought it was hilarious when my friend Amy brought over Barbie dolls for the girls and L snatched her own new Barbie along with Jaz's, and raced them to the kitchen where she promptly shaved both their heads. What always fascinated me was their lack of overt jealously or competition with one another, as if having such different personalities gave them a bye. They'd bicker like crazy, but they didn't feel the need to compete, only the need to support and protect. And in the years to follow, when times got tough, no one cheered harder for Jaz or protected her more vehemently than L.

The summer L was five, I was in the market for a new car, so I took her and Jaz to the dealership so they could sit in the backseats of dif-ferent models and test them out. L really wanted me to get a minivan.

To a five-year-old, a big comfy car with TV screens in the back seemed idyllic. I was not interested. I had vowed to never drive a minivan.

"Mom, you should get a minivan. It would be so much fun."

"I'm not getting a minivan. One day you'll get it; I'm too cool to drive a minivan. I just can't do it," I said.

"Please."

"I'll tell you what. If I get a minivan, I'm going to keep it for 11 years, and when you're 16 I'll give it to you for you to drive."

"Awesome," she squealed. "I'll paint it black with big flames on the sides and put a mattress in the back and speakers all over. It'll be amazing." "We're not getting a minivan," I said.

That same summer L went to Banner Day Camp for the first time. To say I was nervous that first day as she boarded the bus full of kids she didn't know would be an understatement. I had learned that it took her a while to get used to new things, and first days were often difficult—for *both* of us. I kept my workday light, knowing it would be tough to concentrate, and began waiting on the driveway for the bus to return about an hour before it was scheduled back. I wanted to play it safe and didn't want to risk the bus pulling up and my not being there.

At about 4:15 that afternoon, I heard the hulking sounds of the Crazy Cow Bus turning onto our street. All of the Banner buses had names, and ours was the Crazy Cow. I put on my best happy face, trying to hide my nerves from L, not knowing what kind of mood she'd be in. The doors to the bus opened, and she bounded up the driveway as if she had a rocket on her back. She was beaming! Her smile took up her whole face, and she was talking a mile a minute.

I had never seen her show such passion for something; on the surface, she shouldn't have really liked it. Being away from home with a bunch of other kids, doing organized activities that are designed for typical five-year-old's?

None of that should have appealed to L's personality, yet she loved it. There was something about the energy there that let L not only be a kid, but actually revel in being a kid. It was magical for her, and she spent seven summers there. She would have kept going had her body allowed her to.

That first summer she learned that each bus prepared a bus song that they would perform at Banner-amma on stage for the whole camp. The Crazy Cow bus song that year was to the tune of the Back Street Boys' "Everybody." The lyrics *Everybody, rock your body, yeah yeah* were replaced with *Everybody, milk your udders, moo moo*. L would come home singing, "*Milk your udders, moo moo,*" and we would just about fall over laughing. The best part for L was that, at the eleventh hour, the Crazy Cow bus song was banned for being inappropriate. This was perhaps the funniest thing L had ever heard. Far better than performing the bus song was *not* performing the bus song because of its inappropriate lyrics.

When L was five and a half, Disney released the prequel to *The Little Mermaid* on DVD. It explains how King Triton came to be such a grumpy old curmudgeon of a merman. Like all good Disney movies, it depicts the tragic death of Ariel's mom in the first scene. L sat next to Jaz, who had just turned four, as they watched the movie, munching on sourdough toast and chicken nuggets. About halfway through, Jaz looked up and realized there was no mom. "Where's the mom?" she asked innocently. L turned to her sister, placed her hands on her wrists, looked her in the eye, and very matterof-factly said, "The mom is dead, Jaz. She got smooshed by a boat in the beginning of the movie. Get over it."

Parents often feel a sense of bittersweet melancholy when they realize a child has lost her innocence. There is a simplicity to childhood that we want to hold forever, even though rationally we know it's impossible. I used to joke that L was born without innocence, so she never had it to lose.

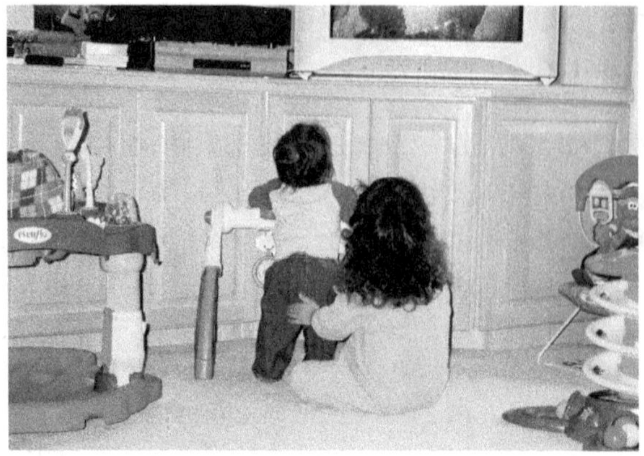

L, age 2, taking care of Jaz, age 7 months, 2005.

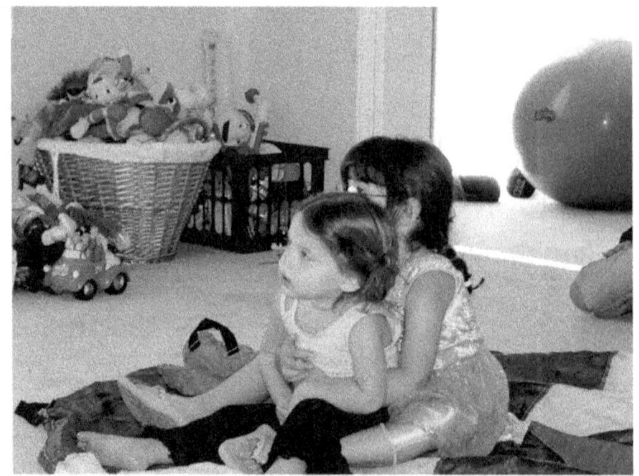

L, age 3 and Jaz, age 1½, 2006.

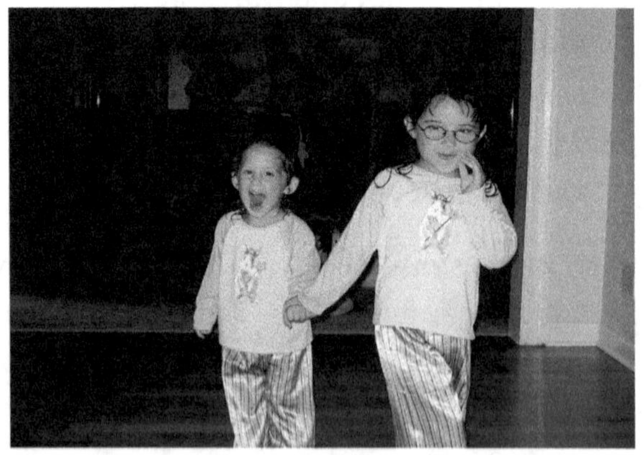

L, age 3½ and Jaz, age 2.

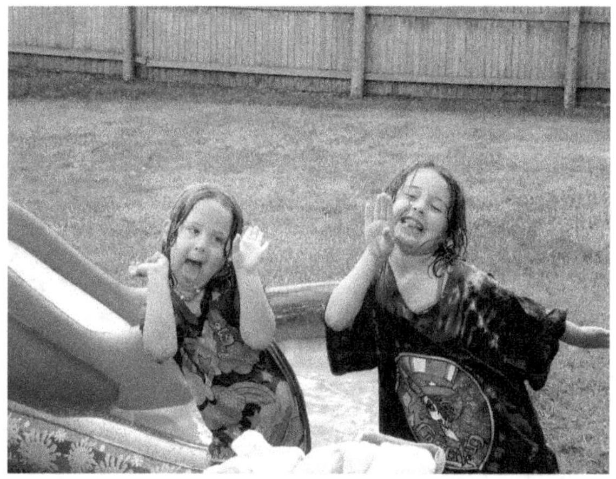

L, age 4½ and Jaz, age 3.

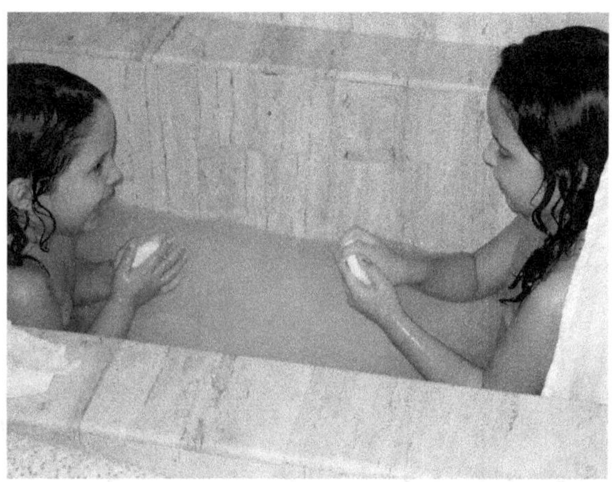

Bath time, L, age 4½ and Jaz, age 3.

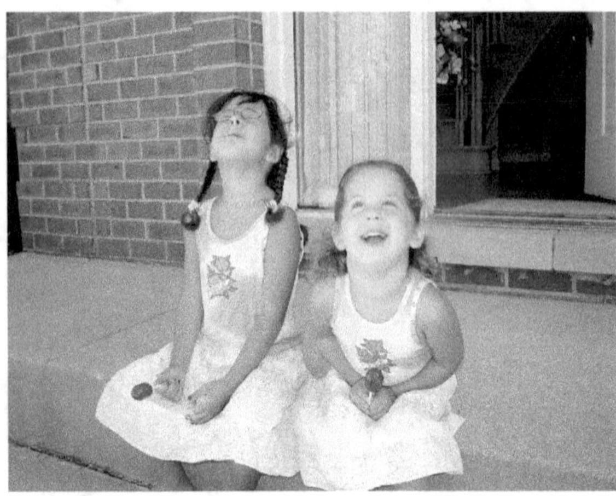

Jaz's third birthday with L, age 4½, July 12, 2007.

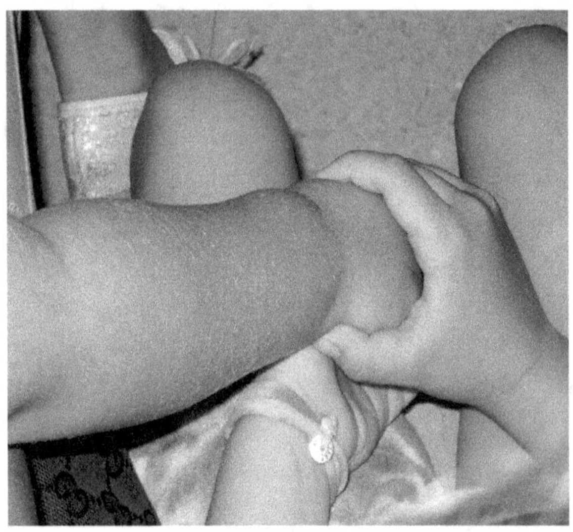

*L holding her sister's hand at Jaz's preschool graduation, 2009.
L, age 6 and Jaz age 4½.*

2009 (age 6)

L had complained of headaches on and off since she was quite young, but by age six or seven, the headaches had turned into full-blown migraines. They didn't come very often, but when they did, she was down for the count. Both my mom and sister had suffered from migraines, so I wasn't surprised, but I certainly wanted to bring her some relief. The pediatrician L saw at the time was pretty dismissive. "Kids don't get migraines. They are probably just headaches. She's calling them migraines, but they're not." The thing is, they were.

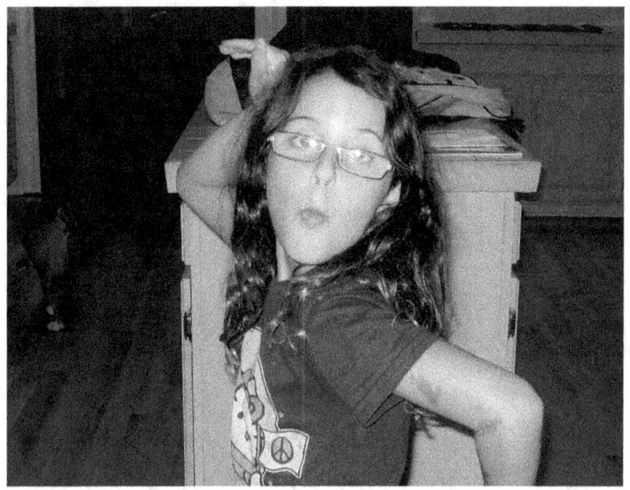

L in one of her signature poses, age 6.

Summer 2010 (age 7)

Every summer I would try to take the girls on a short vacation before the school year started. We had a tradition of going to Arizona in August. I love the heat, the girls would be in the pool all day, and the Four Seasons would practically pay us to go there! It worked for us. In August of 2010, as we were preparing to head to the lap of luxury, a friend of mine whose daughter had been friends with L since preschool called and asked if we wanted to join her family at Family Camp at a camp in Michigan. At the end of their regular overnight camp session for girls, they open the camp to families. She raved about how much fun it was. Each family got their own cabin, and you got to spend a week at camp waterskiing, horseback riding, eating in the mess hall, the works!

For some reason we decided to go, playfully cursing them as we were packing towels, bedding, bug repellent, etc. instead of heading to the Four Seasons. When we got to Family Camp, our friends were nice enough to loan us their broom and mop to clean the cabin (they were experienced; we were clearly novices). Jaz, who had just turned six, was in heaven. She made her bed with her Hello Kitty comforter and proudly declared that when she was old enough, this is where she wanted to go to overnight camp. It would become Jaz's happy place, and she would spend eight summers there. L was more ambivalent. The whole communal-living thing didn't sit really well with her, and she was definitely not a fan of the mess hall. But she did discover the horses and, when she was riding, she was happy.

True to camp form, there was an evening activity each night. It was perhaps the second or third night that the evening activity was a talent show. Kids of all ages took the stage to dance and jump around. Jaz did five perfect cartwheels. Then L took the stage. In front of 100 people, she started singing Journey's "Don't Stop Believin'" a cappella. After the first verse, the whole camp was signing along with her, the collective energy in the pavilion palpable. I'm not sure if L ever really knew what she did that night. I don't know if she realized how the power of her presence alone brought people together. For those of us who were there, it was unforgettable.

Don't stop believin', hold on to that feeling...

Eight years later, on July 27, 2018, L's memorial service began with the synagogue's cantor singing an acoustic version. *Don't stop believin', hold on to that feeling...*

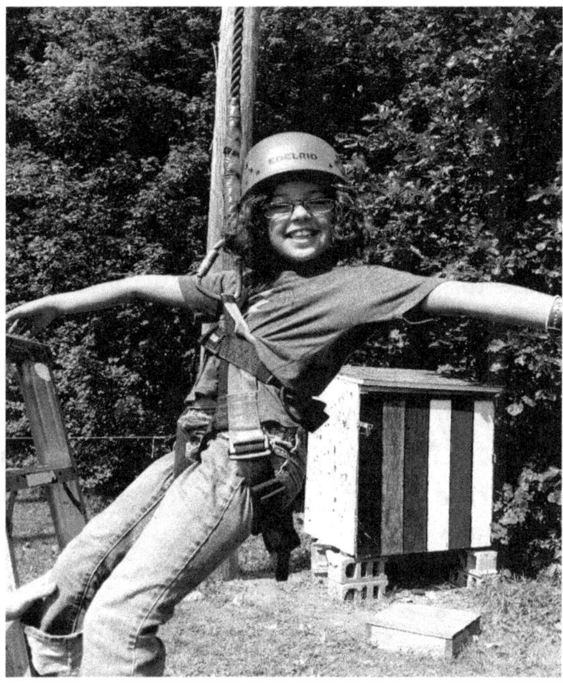

L at Family Camp, 2010, age 7.

2010–2012 (age 7–10)

L loved animals. Farm animals, mostly. She couldn't get enough. Cows, chickens, pigs, goats—and frogs—she always loved frogs. Every year for Hanukkah, my mom would "buy" her a goat or a cow from the Heifer Foundation to support those in need. She totally appreciated the quirkiness of her Grandma Bobbie. Her grandma was notoriously frugal and was becoming more eccentric by the day. One evening when we were having dinner at her grandma's, L noticed a yogurt in the fridge that had expired two years prior. With this, she hatched an idea. She made name tags for herself, Jaz, and her Auntie D, that read "Inspector." The three of them then proceeded to raid every cupboard, every inch of the freezer, and the refrigerator at Grandma Bobbie's, looking for expired food. They found mustards and capers that were 20 years old, meats in the freezer that were 12 years old, salad dressings that were nine years old. She roared with gleeful laughter, discovering things that were older than she. The older something was, the harder she laughed. "Inspector" would become one of L and Jaz's favorite games to play with their grandma.

She dabbled with sports. L was a strong swimmer, earning lifeguard status at Banner by age seven, her counselor cheering her on from the side as she passed the final test of rescuing a brick from the bottom of a 12-foot pool. She joined a swim team but eventually gave it up. Her coaches would criticize her for hyperextending her elbows and shoulders with every stroke. "I can't help it," she would say. "This is just how my arms go." I didn't think much of it at the time. She tried soccer too. But after twisting her ankles several times in one season, she gave that up as well. She seemed to twist her ankles easily. It was not uncommon for her to spend a weekend with a quick x-ray in the ER and her ankle wrapped in an Ace bandage. At the time, I didn't think much of that either.

L started second grade in the fall of 2010. She was a voracious learner who would dig into topics with such depth that it left most adults wondering how on earth she knew so much, where she went to research topics, and how she could retain so much information about so many things. When she was older, she would express frustration over the fact that she knew she could not possibly learn everything she wanted to learn in her lifetime—because she literally wanted to learn everything. Her second-grade teacher Linda became one of the most important people in her life (and mine). She became L's confidante, and one of my closest friends. She understood L, was fascinated by her, and knew that L was here to teach her as much as she was here to teach L.

She encouraged L to research anything and everything she was interested in.

She talked to L about her spirituality (she was one of the few people in whom L confided that she could connect with spirits), and she embraced L not as an eight-year-old, but as a soul who was timeless and ageless. When the school year ended, L wanted to get Linda something special. She found an adorable stuffed animal, a cow, and ordered one for herself and one for Linda so that they would always be connected (like I said, she always had a thing for farm animals). Her cow's name was Grazer. He would be L's permanent companion for the next seven years, with her at every hospital stay, waiting for her whenever the fog of anesthesia began to clear, and comforting her when she took her last breath.

Linda encouraged L to submit her poetry to a local poetry competition. L did and won honorable mention. At the ceremony one of the judges told me that the reason she did not win first prize was that no one actually believed that the poem was written by an eight-year-old. I assured the judge that she wrote it completely on her own. Here it is.

Nipula

L Grey

January 30, 2011 (age 8)

It cannot be life
Of the vibrations they come
Over a force they leap and twirl
Many rise, many pray
No, no, God, we're OK.
Leave the creatures of earth at their own level
They will rise to only the vibrations of love
When time ends.

I've read this poem hundreds of times since she first wrote it at age eight. But it was only after her death that I wondered what she really meant by "vibrations." What did she know? What was she saying? What was she trying to tell us?

L could never spell. It was kind of a joke between us. Here was the brilliant child who could barely spell the word *the*. By third grade she told me that when she read, the words were blurry and jumped around on the page. She had worn glasses since she was 18 months old, so my first step was to check her prescription. Her glasses were fine. I then got her a complete neuropsychological workup with a lovely psychologist I had known since kindergarten. The results were fascinating. L was off the charts in her cognition, but her visual processing, her ability to make sense of symbols, was in the first percentile.

The psychologist recommended vision therapy to help train her brain to process symbols. L spent the bulk of third grade going to vision therapy once a week to improve her visual processing. At the end of nine months her visual processing was in the 65th percentile. She had worked hard. The school had not. Despite the psychologist's recommendations that the school provide services to accommodate L being twice exceptional (meaning exceptionally gifted in one area and deficient in another), the school refused. They told us they would either offer her gifted services or special assistance services to address the visual processing, but not both. I chose the gifted services and bought her a kindle. I would order all her books online, and she could then increase the font to a size that was comfortable for her. That seemed to do the trick. It was a novel idea at the time.

During this period L continued to write poetry. Some of it was dark, some whimsical. All of it was beyond her years and, in retrospect, seemed to foreshadow a deep, unexplainable knowing that L had. As I re-read every word she ever wrote, I finally began to understand what L's truth had been all along. She had one foot in this world, and one foot in another. Somewhere deep in her soul she knew she was not meant to be here for long. She knew her home was somewhere else, and she did not fight or fear it. She knew her soul would live on. L wrote these poems three and a half years before she got sick, seven years before she died.

Untitled

L Grey

August 22, 2011 (age 8)

With every day must come a dusk
With every night must come a dawn
For every angel and every devil has their own sort of way.
So, when I float up to the sky
Please sing to me
Just the way I sing to you
One note at a time.
I'm telling you please listen so
Every angel, every devil, has their own sort of way
For every dusk must come a night
And in that night I shall float all the way up into the clouds we look upon
And when I do please do not fight it
Just sing to me the way I sing to you
One note at a time.

Steam

L Grey

September 27, 2011 (age 8)

Every day the sun must set below the mountain tops
For then a dark cloud of steam must fill the air and love it dear
I do not know
But I have chosen to fight
Do not bring the peace home yet
For it is fake
And I have chosen to fight
For I am a girl of pride
And winning is not on my side

Wind- Ter
L Grey
September 30, 2011 (age 8)

The winds will break the house of shelter
And right then you will be fine
But as it goes on
Your vibrations will lie in the hands of others
And when you go up to the sky
A peaceful place where souls may cry
Tears of joy, tears of sorrow
They'll be with you
And sometime when I grow up
Your soul will take part in those with none
So let the winds holler
I'll come, I will, I will.

On November 10, 2012, two days shy of her tenth birthday, and two and a half years before the CRPS began, L wrote this about fiery, burning pain.

Free to Rage
L Grey
November 10, 2012 (two days shy of age 10)

A yellow light, too hot for pain
Rotting my heart away.
No, not that.
It only pumps steaming blood through my rigid veins.
My head, it does though, burning in fire, hot and red
Rage in my eyes to anger the witch
To scream, to kick, to punish all near, close
Will condemn me more to suffer this day, this world
To avert my gaze—nice, it is, but I can't
I must stay to live again, to finish
If only I could swallow my soul

Only time will tell what will be done
But for now, life, hotter than sun.

Two months later, and five and a half years before her death, she wrote these:

Black Butterfly
L Grey
January 30, 2013 (age 10)

Death, a five letter word to scare most all,
But it is bliss, sweet, sweet bliss to live on.
So why would you hate it? The change, the concept,
Well death is the black butterfly.
In a sea of white, so attractive,
But why would you ever surrender to beauty?
Oh no, you must fit in, you will fit in
Just know this, while you shake with rigid fear,
I'll grow, blossom.
Leave this madness to comfort.
So go on, shoo the black butterfly.
It will fly around soon enough

Heavens & Guns
L Grey
January 30, 2013 (age 10)

I sit here now, examining the tear stained eyes that are examining me back.
I look at the girl in which you would think the black clothes would keep her
so well hidden in this dark world, but in fact, they do the opposite. I swear
quietly before closing my eyes, so I can take off my skin, then open them
'cause the blood should not bother me, I can't be a healer if I'm scared of it.
I begin to walk to the ladder to go home, but it just keeps moving far-
ther and farther away. Once again, I'm mortified when I snap back into
reality; what I really want to do is travel back to my popped bubble,
blow it up, and hop in to go home.

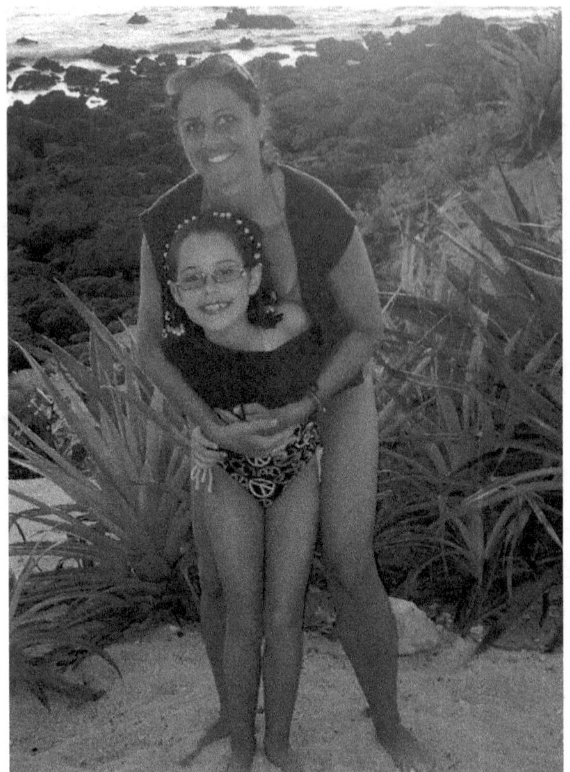

L and me when she was 7.

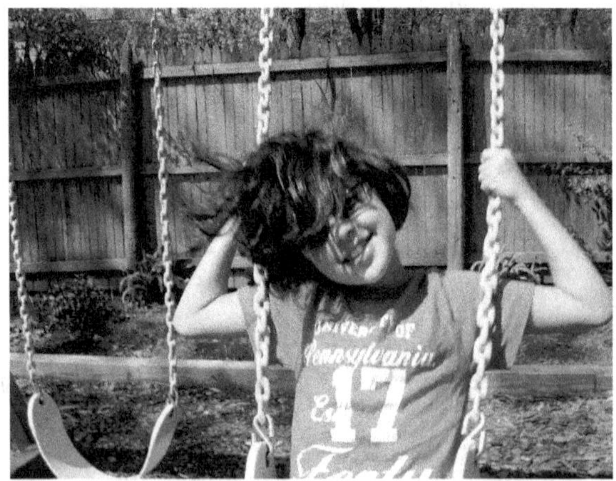

L age 8.

2012 (age 9)

L began fourth grade that fall, and while she had been lucky with teachers who, to that point, were able to nurture her insatiable curiosity, her luck ran out that year. Her teacher was nice enough but could not keep pace with L, and the gifted services the school offered were not sufficient. In the spring of fourth grade, while in Colorado over spring break, we made the decision to transfer L to a gifted school. She began as soon as we returned.

Academically, she was finally home. She continued to write. She wanted her voice out there, yet she was also fiercely private. She created a blog under the pseudonym "Raven" (she would later change this to Grey), since that's the name she thought I should have given her. "L is too feminine," she would say. "Raven is dark and mysterious. It's a much more fitting name for me." Even at age nine, there were precious few things about L that were truly youthful, but her love for her stuffed animals was one. She made no apologies for her attachment to Grazer, and he slept with her every night. Every once in a while, there were other flashes of childhood innocence. She loved sour spray candy and would laugh hysterically when I would try it and frantically search for water to get the taste out of my mouth. I remember taking L and Jaz to see the *Glee* movie. We were sitting in the back row, and at one point, the cast performed a rendition of Pink's "Raise your Glass." L stood up from her chair, and in the back of the theater started dancing with reckless abandon. She would later be embarrassed, and I would forget about it altogether until after her death, when the memory came back with full force at the end of a Soul Cycle class.

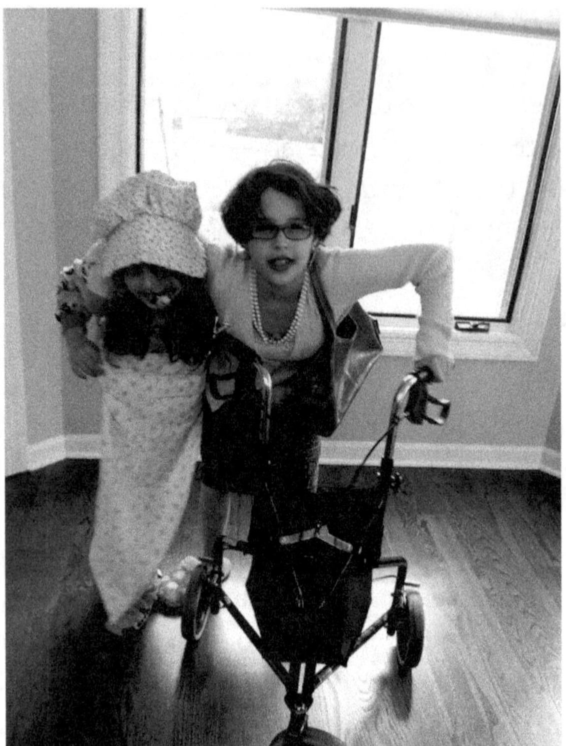

L (age 9) and Jaz, Halloween 2012. Jaz was a baby, L an old lady.

April 2013 (age 10)

"Hey, Momma?" L asked, "What would you say if I told you I liked girls? I mean, not just as friends... you know?"

"L," I said, "I care that you have healthy, loving relationships in your life. Whether you like men or women makes no difference to me. I just want you to have love in your life."

"Ok, good, cuz this isn't like a 'maybe' situation, or an 'experimenting with my sexuality' kinda thing. I'm gay, case closed," she said.

L's coming out was that simple. We sat on her bed and had this conversation, and the whole thing couldn't have taken more than five minutes. I can't say that I was surprised, but I couldn't articulate why.

There was just something about her unique style and unapologetic stance for being true to herself that made it seem almost a given that she would not be straight, as if being straight were far too mundane for her.

It was right around that time that Macklemore released the song "Same Love." Jaz, who was eight at the time, never questioned L's sexual orientation and never felt embarrassed or ashamed that her sister was gay. It was just the opposite. Jaz simply knew L as L, and she accepted and celebrated her for who she was without question. When "Same Love" would come on the radio, Jaz would smile and sing along, proudly exclaiming, "That's my sister!"

As L got older, and especially after she got sick, her sexuality became a more prominent part of her identity and served as the engine that drove her passion for equality and social justice. She would educate us all on gay icons and pioneers of human rights in the LGBTQ community. We learned about the trials and tribulations of Oscar Wilde, her favorite writer, and the significance of the green carnation to the gay community. She'd invariably make us laugh, as she would find a way to turn every story, current event, or historical fact into a lesson about why "the gays" were simply superior to everyone else.

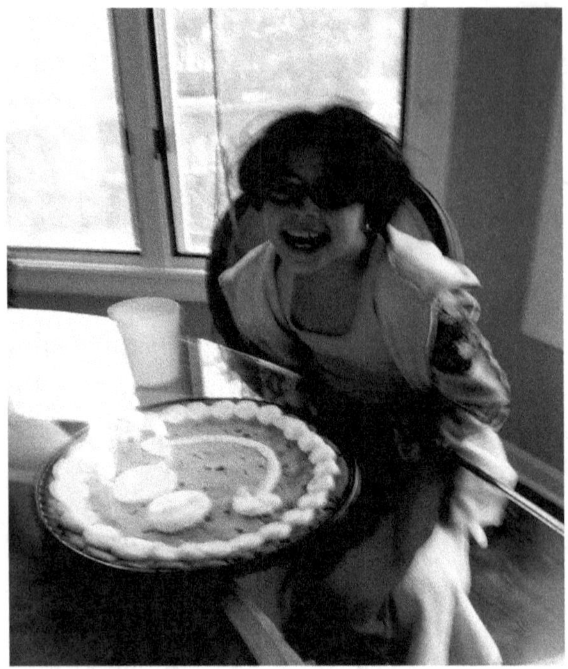

L's 10th birthday, November 12, 2012.

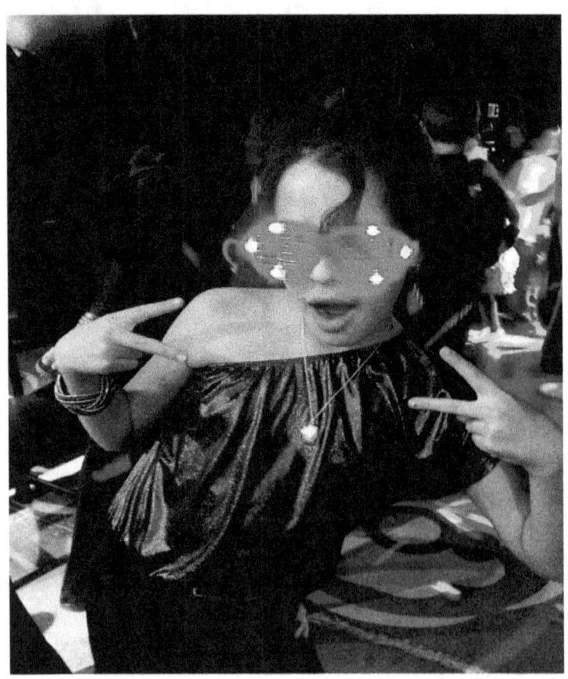

L, age 10.

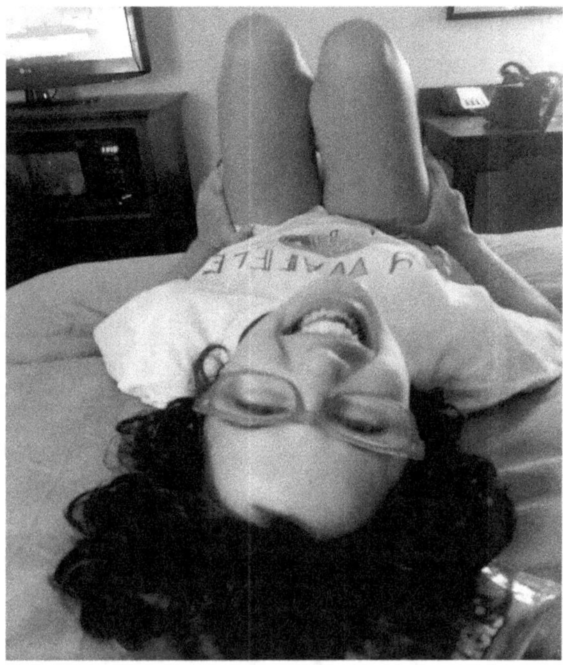

L on a road trip with "D" at age 10.

July 2013 (age 10)

L never enjoyed being too far from home. She would feel a powerful, melancholic homesickness, even when we were on vacation. And yet, she had a desire to see the world, and by this point, at age 10, she was determined to move on from her fear. Her younger sister was planning on spending her first summer at camp in Michigan, as she had planned three years prior. L decided she would go to camp too, but not the same one as her sister. She wanted to go somewhere where there wouldn't be other kids from the neighborhood. She wanted to get away from suburban Chicago.

We researched, and we landed on Camp Birchwood in northern Minnesota. My sister had gone there as a girl and loved it. My sister and L shared a sense of quirkiness, and we thought it would be a good fit. We talked to the camp director who assured us they would keep a good eye on L. She was going to go for 12 days. We looked at the website often, dreamed about what it would be like, planned how she would spend her days, looked at sample menus, and thought about what her favorite meals would be. But she was clearly nervous.

"L," I said, "you know camp is a 'want to' not a 'have to.' You don't have to go."

"But I do have to go, Momma. There is so much I want to do, and all of it requires being away from home. So, I figure, if I can conquer this fear, then I can do anything. It opens up the whole world for me." I couldn't argue with that logic.

Right before she left, L dyed her hair bright blue. This began a trend for her of dying her hair as a form of self-expression. At the airport, as she and the other kids gathered and the camp director introduced himself and assured us the girls would be in good hands, the edginess of L's blue hair stood in sharp contrast to the fear in her eyes. But she was determined, and with watery eyes she followed the group through security and made her way through O'Hare to fly to Minneapolis.

Camp Birchwood posts pictures at the end of each day so that curious, worried parents can look at their girls and reassure themselves that they are okay. There is an anxious anticipation that first night while parents wait for pictures to be posted. When they came in, I saw a photo of L. She was wearing white Bermuda shorts that came down to her knees and an emerald green fleece sweatshirt. She was standing with her cabin, her mouth open wide in what many would mistake for a smile—but which I knew was not. When L was little, she had a fake smile that she would put on for pictures when she needed to. She would open her mouth wide like she was catching raindrops on her tongue. It was cute, and it was fake, and it was what she was doing in this picture at camp.

"Something isn't right," I said, "that's her fake smile."

When I went to overnight camp as a kid, our only means of communication was snail mail. But in 2013 things were different. There were bunk notes: for a dollar you can send an email that gets printed and delivered to your daughter the next morning. For another dollar, you can order special paper, and your child can write a letter that gets scanned and emailed back to you. So, instead of waiting four or five days for communication, you can communicate within 24 hours. I immediately sent L a bunk note asking how she was liking camp and telling her that I paid for special paper, so she could write me back and I'd get it the very next day. At 10:00 am the next morning, I received her first bunk note.

HELP ME. PLEASE HELP ME. YOU NEED TO GET ME OUT OF HERE. THIS IS NOT HOMESICKNESS. PLEASE, MOMMA, PLEASE HELP ME.

It would not have surprised me if L had been homesick and had not enjoyed overnight camp. I was expecting that. But I also knew L, and she was incredibly self-aware. Something about this didn't feel like straight-up homesickness. I immediately called camp and asked to talk to the director. They told me the director was at the waterfront and assured me that I would get a call back later in the day. I told them about the bunk note and about my concerns. "Yes, she's a little homesick," the woman on the phone said, "but she is easily distracted. She should be fine." That was my next clue. L was many things, but easily distracted was not one of them.

After making several more attempts to reach the director, I finally heard back that evening and was told the same thing, "She's easily distracted." That night, as Jaz and I sat at dinner, I contemplated my next move. Jaz, who was eight at the time, said "I don't know why you are even talking about this. You should go get her right now." I decided if the next day's bunk notes had the same tone, we would go straight to Minnesota. At 10:00 the next morning, my email was filled with seven bunk notes from L. All said basically the same thing.

PLEASE, PLEASE, PLEASE, HELP ME. I CAN'T STAY HERE.

It struck me that some counselor was responsible for scanning these notes. Surely someone must have seen her pleas in all capitals, yet no one there seemed alarmed. We went straight to the airport, caught the next flight to Minneapolis, rented the last car they had (a badass Ford 150, one of the few moments of comic relief in the ordeal) and drove to LaPorte, Minnesota, where we got L with barely a goodbye to the director and started the journey home. I held L in a deep embrace. After putting her to bed upon her arrival home, I said to myself, "Something happened; she has PTSD." It did not require the PhD I have in psychology to determine that.

In the days that followed, L was noticeably relieved to be home, and when I asked her what had happened, she described a place that was clearly not emotionally safe. She talked about counselors who were absent, she talked about asking to talk to the director's wife and being denied access, she talked about wandering off in the woods by herself, with no one noticing, where she would quietly have panic attacks. There was no doubt bringing her home was the right thing. She made it clear she was not comfortable there. She did not say anything more.

September 2013 (age 10)

L was depressed, and she knew it. Academically she was thriving. Her new school provided the challenges she craved, and she had teachers who delighted in her curious nature, humor, and insight. But she was depressed. I reached out to a former professor of mine, a kind-hearted and compassionate psychologist, and asked if she would work with L. She agreed. After their first meeting, she met with me to share her observations.

"Has she ever been abused?" she asked.

I was shocked. "No, I can't think of a situation in which she would have been abused; she's never been in the care of anyone other than immediate family," I said.

"I am not saying she has been, but I am telling you she presents like someone who has been sexually abused."

Two years later, as L's illness was burning her alive, my shock would turn to rage, heartbreak, and helplessness when I finally learned the truth.

2014 (age 11)

L was in fifth grade, and at the time there seemed to be a relative calm in her world. It was her first full year at her new school, and she was settling in, navigating the mysterious and complex world of being a gay, gifted, middleschool girl. She had her dark moments, for sure, but they were not unexpected. L was never a lighthearted, happy-go-lucky kid, and the social pressures of middle school didn't make things any lighter. But her therapy seemed to be helping, and even in her darker moments she never questioned who she was. She held onto her identity and her truth with steadfast conviction. L was always vocal and opinionated, almost from birth, so it was no surprise that as she entered adolescence her voice became louder and her opinions stronger and better informed by data. She and my dad would get into heated philosophical debates on whether respect for elders should be automatically granted or whether it needed to be earned. She started thinking about societal ills like institutional racism and infrastructures designed to keep poor people marginalized.

Her courage continued to grow, and while in Florida that year, she decided to come out to her grandpa. We were sitting at dinner when, completely out of nowhere, she just blurted out, "Hey, I'm gay." My dad's reaction was priceless, and classic Dad: "Thank goodness," he laughed. "At least I don't have to worry about you marrying a terrorist, 'cuz I can't think of any female terrorists; they're all guys. Thank you, L. Now I can scratch that worry off my list!"

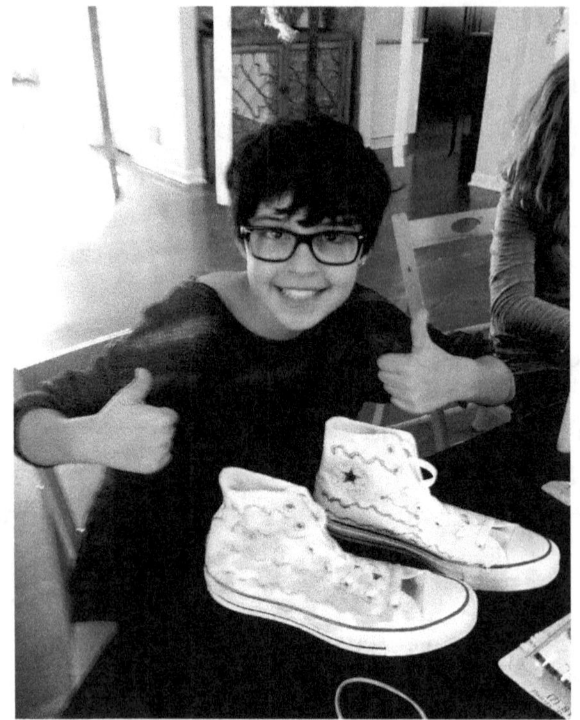

L's 11th birthday, November 12, 2013.

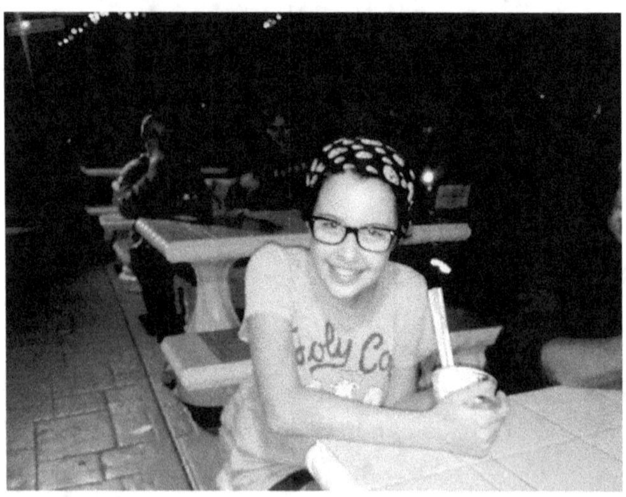

L in Sanibel, December 2014, her last healthy trip there.

January–April 2015 (age 12, before CRPS)

L seemed to be finding her groove. She was doing well in school, her psychotherapy seemed to be going well, and she seemed far more upbeat. There was a paradox to L. She was, at times, dark, serious, and brooding and at other times so ridiculously funny, she would have us all in stitches. She was particularly good at impressions. She had her uncle's elevator pitch for his business down pat, including the exact grip of his handshake. She could imitate my dad when he was upset with me, asking, "Uh, Vishy (his nickname for me), could we have a chit-chat?"

Our favorite one was of Barbara, the elderly woman at the Robert Crown Center for Health Education where she and her classmates took a field trip to fulfill the mandatory sex ed requirement. "Ladies," L would say in a slow drawl, "you shove the tampon into your vaginal canal, like I'm doing on this mannequin. Let me repeat, you shove the tampon into your vaginal canal. Any questions?" I'd be laughing so hard I'd have to cross my legs to keep from having an accident. "There's no shoving," I would remind both girls, "There should be no reason to shove anything, ever." "I'm feelin' you now, Mr. Krabs," L would say. We'd laugh even harder.

She would wonder aloud what her path in adulthood would be. Would she go to medical school and become a neurosurgeon? (She had always been fascinated by the brain.) Would she go to law school and become a social justice advocate? Would she be a literature professor at a liberal arts college, living a bohemian lifestyle with her wife and some chickens or goats? Would she write for *Saturday Night Live*? She would have thrived at all of it. A good problem to have, we would joke, to have so many options.

L decided to audition for the youth ensemble at The Second City to explore the whole improv/*SNL* path. There were hundreds of kids auditioning for two spots. L was the youngest by two to three years. She got one of the spots. These kids were funny and smart; they wrote their own sketches and cast them on their own, performing new ones every few months in Second City's Black Box Theater to a packed house. Many in the troupe had been performing together for years, and L wondered how she would fit in with them, but they welcomed her readily.

In between rehearsals they headed down to Starbucks or Chipotle, where they would sip coffee and munch on chips in the delighted way teenagers do when they are on the brink of adulthood, their whole lives stretching before them. There was a healthy competition, as they would try to outdo each other with sarcastic jokes and pop-culture references. L was comfortable hanging out with these kids who were several years older, and they were comfortable with her. It made sense. She was an old soul who could never quite relate to kids her own age. With this troupe, probably for the first time in her life, she felt like she belonged.

Once she became sick she could no longer perform, but she always wanted to go back when she was better, and her troupe never forgot her.

I received this beautiful note from one of her castmates shortly after she died.

Dear Vanessa

I am writing to you to express my sincere condolences for the passing of L. I just wanted to take my time to tell you what a strong, brilliant, and exceptional person she was. She was never defined by her shortcomings, although I cannot remember any at all. I knew L when we were both younger and worked together in the youth ensemble at Second City; she was twelve when I was fourteen, but I knew potential when I saw it.

She was an exceptional writer in our sketch comedy performances, and I actually had the privilege to bring one of her best sketches to the stage. I still remember her "Puberty" scene as being the wittiest and funniest thing I had read and was always eager to see how she'd top herself. Not surprising, she always did, never failing to get a laugh from the audiences. A few of my best memories with her were sitting on the steps outside of class talking about pop culture; I had not met anyone with such a well-rounded knowledge on every topic I could bring up. She could best be described as a savant and a true inspiration to others within the organization, never ceasing to make new friends and be a fantastic influence on everyone.

When I first heard about her diagnosis, I was heartbroken to hear that she would not return to Second City. She once told me she would try to audition again, wheelchair or not. She told me she would audition, going so far as making a pun saying, "I'm a transformer that broke halfway through." Dark humor as it may seem, she was always funny, and that's how I love to remember her. Over time we began to grow apart, as many tend to do when living far away, but I always hoped to visit and work with her again. We always viewed her as part of our little unconventional family at Second City. We were all deeply saddened to hear of her passing but take solace in the fact that we got to meet such an amazing person. I will never meet a more tenacious, thoughtful, and hilarious person in my life, but I'm okay with that.

All because I got to know L. Grey.

Part II: During

April 21, 2015 (age 12)

L was 12 years old and in sixth grade. She was thriving academically, creating the unique bonds with her favorite teachers, as she was prone to do. She would spend lunches with her English teacher discussing their favorite books. She would pop in to see her Social Studies teacher whose bold, unapologetic, and unconventional style struck a deep chord within L. She would stay after school with her math teacher, a woman whose serious exterior intimidated many but whose compassionate core was there for those who were bold enough to get to know her. It didn't hurt that she and L shared the same sarcastic sense of humor and impatience with most other people.

L had just finished a monthlong series of performances with Second City. Her dark humor and impeccable sense of comedic timing brought the house down in her last performance. Two days after the show wound down, L came home from school and casually mentioned that she had twisted her ankle while jumping off a ledge during recess. She wasn't in pain, and there was no swelling or bruising; it was a passing comment. At 5:00 the next morning she called me in her room.

"Something is wrong, Mom," she said. "My leg is on fire. It's like it has been dunked in lighter fluid and someone is holding a blow torch to it."

I looked at her leg, and while there was no swelling and she had full range of motion, her skin was turning different shades of purple and red as we sat there talking. She was unable to put any pressure on her foot, so I carried her to the car, we headed to the ER, and I carried her in. The x-rays revealed no injury, and the ER doctors were perplexed. They sent us home with crutches and a referral to see an orthopedic surgeon. It was two days before they could get her in, and her grandma took her so that I could go to work. My phone sat beside me during my meetings as I awaited the news. The text came at around 3:00 pm.

"L has something called complex regional pain syndrome," it said. "The orthopedic is referring us to a doctor at the Rehab Institute of Chicago (RIC), which specializes in this."

"Is it serious? Is the doctor concerned?" I asked.

"The doctor has seen this before, and in children it usually resolves itself in a few weeks," she replied.

I remember thinking *a few weeks?!* The idea of L being in pain for a few weeks... it seemed like an eternity. Little did we know that she would be burning alive, from the inside out, for over three years.

May–June 2015 (age 12)

Complex regional pain syndrome (CRPS) is known as the single most painful condition to afflict humans. That's worth repeating. *CRPS is considered the most painful condition known to humans.*

Although there is no actual injury, the brain sends pain signals to parts of the body, creating the sensation that you are being burned alive. The McGill pain scale, which estimates the pain associated with various injuries and conditions, places CRPS at the top of the stack, above amputation without anesthesia. And the pain never relents. Never. Not for one second.

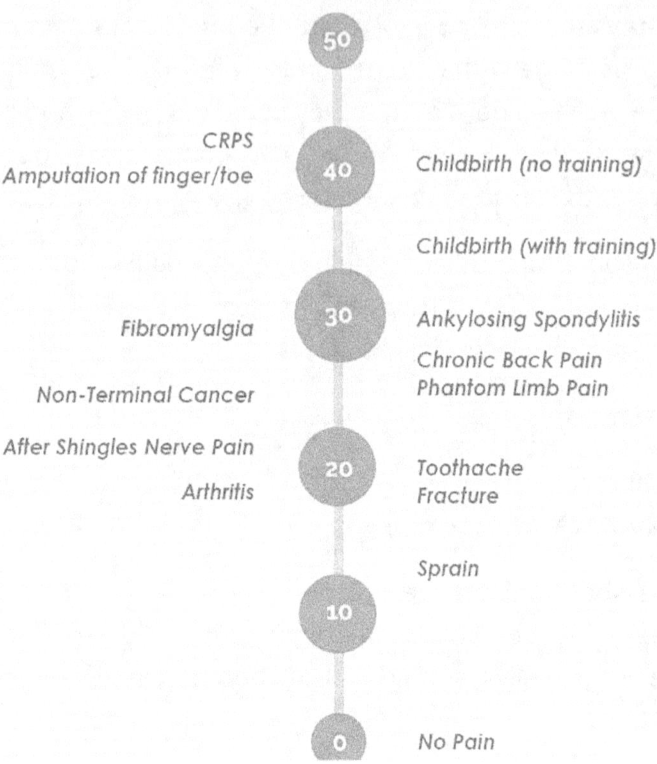

McGill Pain Index Chart

And it spreads. Imagine a moldy strawberry in the middle of a carton of fresh berries. The mold from that first berry quickly spreads to its neighbors, ultimately ruining the whole batch. By May of 2015 L's pain had traveled up her left leg so that everything from her upper thigh down was on fire.

This poem that L wrote over a year into her illness perhaps comes close to describing the pain.

Sand Paper
L Grey
May 26, 2016 (age 13)

Salting raw wounds
Charred muscle
Boiled blood
Bones scraped, drilled, broken
Cemented joints and electric currents

"Good news," the rehab doctor said. "L has been accepted into the intensive physical therapy program at RIC. It's four days a week of physical therapy for four hours a day. The program is eight weeks. It will be intense, but this is the best course of treatment for CRPS."

There goes her summer, I thought, hoping she could still go to Banner for the last few weeks of the season.

L was a trooper. This would come to be her moniker for the next three years. She faced things, endured things that no living soul I know could have endured. And she protected everyone from it. Were it not for her crutches and, in the months to come, her wheelchair, no one would have known that she was suffering. She did not shed a tear. The only thing that betrayed her secret was her eyes, which held a deep, dark, indescribable burden. But you would have to know her well, and you would have to look carefully to even catch a glimpse of it.

She went to physical therapy every day, and she pushed herself hard. The touch of a tissue on her legs felt like razor blades slicing her skin, yet she was determined to try to get her skinny jeans back on. Because her pain was invisible, many people assumed it wasn't that bad, or that she was not working hard enough. "Push harder." "You need a positive attitude." "If the pain is still there, it must be because your attitude isn't right." "Why are you holding onto the pain? Why don't you want to get better?" L heard these remarks on a daily basis. I would come to her defense, tell them they didn't understand and beg them to show her compassion, only to be chided for not pushing her harder myself. In the years to come, these comments became more aggressive, "You're a little shit. You're fucked in the head," some would say. These comments became so detrimental to her that she would cut certain people out of her life. For the moment, however, at age 12, L did her best to grin and bear it.

We learned quickly that spring that the most powerful pain medication could not touch the burning nerve pain. Our pediatrician at the time brought over a topical morphine that his mother-in-law had used in hospice as her cancer consumed her, in the hopes that it might help. Just applying it was torture, as the simplest touch, even from her own hand, was unbearable. Within minutes, the morphine had soaked into her blood stream, and as she downed her sixth piece of sourdough toast (a perennial favorite of hers), she said in between bites, "Don't give this to me again. I'm high as a kite, but I still feel all the pain, so I probably shouldn't ever use this."

Over the course of her illness, I thought often about the single thing that any sick patient, young or old, craves. Pain relief. I thought about what their family members would hold dear. "Please just don't let them suffer." It is so obvious that we don't even really think about it. When someone is in the hospital, we ask doctors, "Is he in pain?" or "Can you give her something to make her more comfortable?" When people approach their final days, and we know the end is near, our singular focus is the alleviation of pain so that they do not needlessly suffer. We give them as much morphine as is legal so that they can have peace because, ultimately, that's what they want and what we want for them.

A heavy enough dose of pain medication would put L to sleep, and in a drug-induced slumber she would sometimes be unaware of the pain. But there was never a *waking* moment when the pain subsided. Never. *Not one.* This was a hard concept for family, friends, and doctors to understand. I stopped giving her the narcotics doctors were so eager to prescribe because they simply would not bring her any waking relief. New doctors would constantly ask what we were doing to manage her pain. "Nothing," I would reply. "It can't be managed. That's the whole problem."

Canvas

L Grey

June 3, 2015 (age 12)

my canvas is colored,
my pencils are dull.
emotions are soaring
life ceases to lull.
my blood may be clean,
but I'm dying from pain
my face drenched with tears,
on my soul is a stain.
physical limits create new rules,
for my fiery heart, and
screaming brain.

Untitled

L Grey

June 3, 2015 (age 12)

I've become a black dot
in a sea of white-
surrounded by red.
im alone, no dots in sight-
but inside i have my red.
i built a black fence, to keep out the red,
but instead, I'm alone.
i built it too close to home.
I've become a red dot,
in a see of black.
nothing in sight
and flickering out, the last shred of will.

June 22, 2015, 12:07 am (age 12)

When the CRPS began I started sleeping with my phone right next to my ear, on full volume, even though I had always been a light sleeper and, once I became a mom, the gentlest cough or sneeze would wake me. But, nevertheless, I kept it on loud. If L needed something, and the pain was too intense for her to call for me or to come get me, she needed to be able to text me.

When you have a sick child, there is no sound worse than the ping of a text coming through in the middle of the night.

Can you come in? the text read.

I entered her room, and she was lying on her stomach, her left leg elevated slightly so that it was not touching the bed. Her whole body was shaking. Earlier that day she had pushed herself hard in physical therapy; she even managed to get a pair of skinny jeans on and texted me a photo. Her teeth were clenched, but the jeans were on. Now, in the middle of the night, the pain spiked and was so exquisite that she could not even rest her leg on the bed. Just that amount of contact was too much for her to bear. She rarely shed a tear, but they flowed freely now as she shook uncontrollably in pain. I thought this spike must be a temporary reaction to the physical therapy and would soon subside. The only thing I could think to do was to bring her to the hospital, where I would beg them to sedate her in the hope that she could sleep it off and at least return to baseline when she woke up.

When we arrived at Lurie Children's Hospital in Chicago, renowned as one of the best children's hospitals in the country, they had no idea what to do. They started by putting her on a Dilaudid drip, despite my insistence that opiates did not help her pain. After the topical morphine experience, some research pointed me toward volumes of articles written about the failure of opiates to address CRPS pain and the very real risk that they actually exacerbated the pain as a result of how they impacted brain chemistry. The residents, unfortunately, knew none of this research. When L's stomach began to hurt so badly that she could not swallow, I instructed her to stop pushing the Dilaudid button. While the doctors insisted that the Dilaudid would not cause stomach pain, I remembered my own experience of being on Oxycontin after a car accident, which told me otherwise. The pain in her legs did not subside, and now the pain in her stomach was increasing. L was an avid researcher. At this point in her illness, she knew more about it than most anybody, and she knew it could spread. She was consumed with fear that it had spread to her stomach and that she would no longer be able to eat. The neurologists spoke in voices that were not as hushed as they thought and talked about this being a case of conversion disorder. L heard every word. She knew exactly what conversion disorder was. She knew the doctors did not believe there was a physiological cause to her pain. And so she lay there in pain, scared, shamed, and wondering if there would ever be a doctor who would believe her—if there would ever be a doctor she could trust.

The only thing they could do was give her Valium to make her sleep, and those moments when she drifted off into a purple haze were blissful, but the pain came roaring back as soon as she awoke.

At 7:00 pm on day two of our stay, a new nurse came in and noticed how difficult it was for L to swallow.

"What's wrong?" she asked.

"Ever since the Dilaudid she has had terrible stomach pain. I told her to stop pushing the button, but the pain has not yet subsided, and the doctors have no idea what is wrong," I said.

"She needs heat, that's why," the nurse said. "Opiate induced stomach pain requires heat."

She brought us a heating pack, and within seven minutes L's stomach pain was gone and she was asking for juice and crackers. It was a small miracle in what would become a blur of failed treatments. But at that moment there was hope that the spread of CRPS had stopped, and there was the human connection that comes when a compassionate nurse takes the time to listen in ways that others in the hospital couldn't or wouldn't. I wish I knew her name. L and I never forgot her.

After two days, the doctors said there was nothing they could do. They sent us home with a prescription for Valium to use in case of emergency. That was it. Her pain had spiked and had reset itself at this new advanced level. L could not have anything touch her leg. She could not wear pants, could not rest her leg on the bed, could not go outside in the wind. RIC wanted her to come back to physical therapy to keep pushing through, but we were not going back there. The aggressive physical therapy had caused this spike, and no one seemed to appreciate just how bad it was.

After we returned home, L and I sat in her room, candles lit and essential oils going in the diffuser in an attempt to just keep her nervous system calm. She'd always liked candles. She started waving her hand back and forth over one of the flames, the way children often do. She took my hand and guided it over the flame, lowering it slowly so that it got closer and closer until reflexively I had to pull away. "That's nothing," she said, looking me straight in the eye. "I don't even feel it, compared to the pain in my legs." She then took her own hand, lowered it to the flame, and held it there, unflinching as the flames licked her palm. "I don't even feel it," she said again. Over the years I would try, with varying degrees of success, to hide my tears from her. It was pointless, really. L and I could communicate without speaking, and she saw the sadness in my eyes whether the tears were there or not. But in that moment, I didn't even try to hide them. They rolled down my cheeks in perfect, salty spheres.

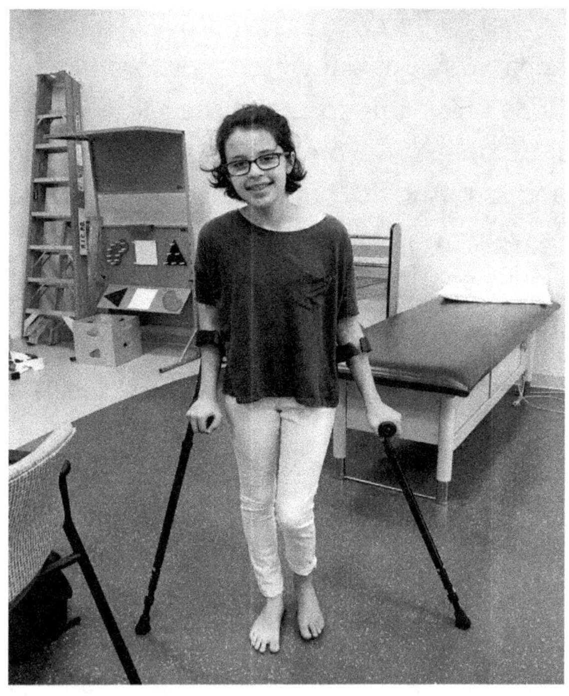

*L in physical therapy, wearing her skinny jeans, June 21, 2015, age 12,
That night, her pain would spike and she wouldn't be able to wear pants*

July 2015 (age 12)

We were in hell. L's pain had spiked and had reset itself, and *absolutely nothing* could touch the pain. Her heart rate was permanently elevated and never dipped below 120. She was on and off Lyrica and Gabapentin. Doctors offered us opiates, which we refused because they didn't work. My kooky, loveable aunt from California brought us medical marijuana—that one helped her sleep and regain her appetite, but in the midst of eating Chex mix with a shovel, L declared it did not help her pain, so maybe it wasn't such a good idea. (We'd later joke that she'd be able to tell her friends that the first time she got high was when she was 12, with her mom).

We went to hypnotists to try to "reset" her brain, traditional Chinese doctors who gave her 52 herbs a day, acupuncturists, and energy healers. In July I got a referral to Dr. Timothy Lubenow, who practiced at Rush and apparently was one of the most prominent specialists in CRPS. I mentioned his name to L, and she said, "Oh, yeah, I've read all his papers. He does some pretty radical stuff with ketamine; you should read about it. And no, I am not going to Mexico or Germany to be put in a seven-day ketamine coma!" I should not have been surprised that L knew so much, but I had no idea what she was talking about. I had never heard of ketamine.

"What's ketamine?" I asked. She gave me *the look.*

"It's known as "special K" on the street. It's a date-rape drug. Actually, it's a horse tranquilizer, but it's used in small doses for anesthesia, and some doctors are using it to treat CRPS. Supposedly, it causes some pretty intense hallucinations."

I had heard of special K (I just didn't know it was actually called ketamine), and it certainly wasn't something I wanted my daughter taking.

"You should look at the research," she chirped. "It's pretty messed up shit. Some doctors fly patients to Germany or Mexico and put them in full-out ketamine comas for a week, and in theory, when they wake up they're better. There's this one case study of a woman who woke up from her coma pain free, but then it came back while she was flying home. So, yeah, I'm not doing that."

She didn't have to convince me of that. No way were we leaving the country for a ketamine coma.

She continued, "Lubenow doesn't do that, but he does three-day infusions where you go in every day for like five hours. He does other things too. I'm not saying I'll for sure do ketamine, but I'll go see Lubenow."

Getting in to see a specialist who has a months-long waiting list is not easy. I called Lubenow's office and was told they had a cancellation the next day, but I would need to provide him with all of her medical records in advance of the appointment, and they weren't sure I would be able to get them. I begged them to give me the time slot and assured them that, one way or another, I would have the medical records from RIC. I learned that obtaining medical records is not a quick process (I thought a simple email would do the trick; I was wrong) and can take up to five weeks. I canceled my meetings for the day, drove downtown to RIC, pleaded with the records department to expedite the process and print me a copy, and left five hours later with hundreds of pages of chart notes.

When we saw Dr. Lubenow, it was clear he knew what he was doing. He understood the pain, the hypersensitivity, the color changes in her skin. He explained the physiology of CRPS. "This will take some time," he said, "probably several months." At the time, several months felt like an eternity. He explained that he had to start with a series of spinal injection blocks, which probably wouldn't work but which insurance needed to see before they would authorize a more promising treatment of a 7–10 day inpatient epidural designed to shut down her central nervous system and reboot it. I asked about ketamine. He said that would only be used if the epidural didn't work. But L was young, and he was hopeful that it would not be necessary.

L spent the remainder of July getting weekly spinal-cord injections, which, not surprisingly, did nothing. I got her a scooter, the kind George Costanza used in Seinfeld, so that she could at least get outside if the wind wasn't too bad. At the end of July, as we were mentally preparing for the inpatient epidural treatment that we knew was inevitable, we decided to go for a scoot. We thought it would be a quick excursion, but we ended up scooting around the neighborhood for hours. There was something L wanted to tell me; that was clear. She was uncharacteristically fumbling for words. She was extremely apologetic and made me promise that I would not be mad at her.

There was something she should have told me a long time ago that she didn't.

She was sorry. I had to promise I wouldn't be mad. This went on for hours. We were home and in her bed by the time she finally found the words.

"Something happened at camp," she cried. "It wasn't consensual. I was raped."

We held each other crying for a long time.

And it made sense. The PTSD when she came home, the depression, and maybe, in some way, we thought, the stress of carrying that secret impacted her nervous system. Maybe, now that she didn't have to carry this secret, her nervous system could quiet down enough and her body could begin to heal. We were hopeful for the epidural.

We would spend the remaining years of L's life unsuccessfully trying to prosecute her abuser. The corruption of local law enforcement in LaPorte Minnesota, the failure to get justice, and the risk he posed to other girls weighed extraordinarily heavy on her heart. As I write this, I am still pursuing justice, and I will not rest until I know other girls are safe. But that is a separate story for another time.

August 1–8, 2015 (age 12)

On August first, after the failed spinal-cord injections, we checked into Rush for the 7–10 day epidural. At minimum, I thought, at least she'd be out of pain for a week and would get a week of respite. The procedure to place the epidural went smoothly, and when L woke from the anesthesia, she had a dreamy smile on her face. "I can't feel my legs," she said. "There's no pain… this might work." I shed one of my few happy tears in that moment, thinking she'd have a week of watching movies in the hospital with no pain while we nervously awaited what would happen when they weaned her off the epidural. The rest of that day was hopeful. As the anesthesia wore off, Dr. Lubenow came into the room filled with promise; he even had L dance, putting pressure on her left leg. We thought we might actually be turning a corner. The hospital chaplain came by to see if L wanted him to lead her in prayer. "I'm a Jewish atheist," she said, "So, yeah, I think I'm good. Thanks, though."

She drifted off to sleep that evening, but at some point in the middle of the night, the efficacy of the epidural started to fail, and her pain came back. She awoke, her mop of magenta hair drenched in sweat, elevating her left leg above the bed, just as she had done all summer. "It's back," was all she said. I didn't understand, could not comprehend how pain could break through an epidural designed to shut down all feeling from the waist down. I knew there was a chance the pain would return once the epidural was stopped, but it never occurred to me that the pain could come back while the epidural was active.

The next seven days were spent with doctors adjusting the dosage in the infusion and coming in to give her boluses of fentanyl. Her leg would slowly drop to the bed as the drug-induced sleep overtook her, and her heart rate would slowly drop, only to spike again later when she awoke, raising her leg off the bed to ease the pain. I would sit and watch the heart-rate monitor for hours. I could tell when she was coming out of sleep because her heart rate would creep up.

On day seven, I remember watching the monitor and noticing that her heart rate was more elevated than it usually was when she was sleeping. I knew something was even more wrong—the pain was starting to break through into her sleep. When she woke up hours later, the pain was so bad she could barely speak. It was clear the epidural wasn't working, and there was no reason for us to be there. There was nothing they could do other than send us home, more frightened and desperate than we had been when we arrived.

September 8, 2015 (age 12)

Ketamine. The thing we dreaded, that we thought was a long shot, that we were assured wouldn't be necessary because surely the CRPS would pass. It was time for ketamine. Doctors and researchers aren't quite sure why ketamine sometimes works. Maybe it is because it has something to do with memory (after all, it is known as a date-rape drug) and makes the brain forget to send these pain signals. Dr. Lubenow had had great success with ketamine. He was confident. Here's how it would work: she would come in for three consecutive days, spending several hours each day getting infused with ketamine. She would be unconscious during the process; propofol guarantees that (this is so that she wouldn't remember any of the crazy hallucinations that ketamine can cause). At the end of each day, once she came to, she would go home, sleep it off, and come back again the next day to do it all over again at an increasingly higher dose of the drug.

Dr. Lubenow cautioned us not to lose faith if L did not have pain relief after day one; the effects build on each other. He likened it to chiseling away at a rock. You make small progress, but you don't see big effects until one final punch causes the whole thing to shatter. The hope was that the ketamine would start to chisel away at the pain and, by the end of day three, the whole pain cycle would shatter.

We arrived at the hospital at 8:00 am for the first round of ketamine. L was two months shy of her 13th birthday. They prepped her with an IV, told me how many milligrams of ketamine she would receive that day, and explained that a resident would be in the room with us the whole time (by law, anyone getting a ketamine infusion needs to be under the direct eye of a physician the whole time). It was after 9:00 when they finally began. L asked that I record her as she was waking up so that she would know what happened and so that she could document it for research. I promised I would. She was asleep within seconds, and I spent the next five hours watching the monitors and massaging and kissing her toes, which could not be touched when she was awake.

I was not sure what to expect when they stopped the infusion and she began to wake up. As the drugs wore off, she began by moving her hands spastically over her face and playing with her lips. She would call out for me and I would hold her hand and rub her head, but it was hard to tell if she knew I was there. Then she began thrashing, her legs banging against the rails of the hospital bed. (Was this hurting her? I wondered but couldn't tell.) She would sit bolt upright in bed, demanding to leave, then fall back down as we held her head so that she did not hurt it against the wall. She would lose bladder function. She would retch violently. She would get bursts of energy and strength, try to do things she physically couldn't, then collapse in a heap.

As she started to talk, her words came out slow and slurred, and the tone of her voice was that of a four-year-old. I would later come to call it her ketamine voice. It was this innocent, childlike voice, but her words were as witty and sharp as they had always been. The contrast was fascinating. And, as she found her words, she would talk—a lot. Over the course of her illness, she would spend a total of 12 days like this. I quickly learned that ketamine was a truth serum for her. She would reveal her inner secrets, her worries, and her burdens, cracking jokes all along the way. But this first time, I didn't know what she would say, and as I recorded her, I assumed much of what she was saying was a hallucination. Later, in the summer of 2018, when I would re-listen to these recordings, I would wonder how much was hallucination and how much was her actual truth.

L: I'm gonna throw up here on earth.

Me: Should I get you a bucket?

L: No, no, no, no... My spaceship is off in the distance. It's already probably further away than the sun. But I'm okay being on earth. I'm just cold.

Me: Want another blanket?

L: I just want pants.

Me: How about another blanket?

L: How about pants? And underwear?

Me: Soon.

L: Soon's not helpful enough.

Me: I know. I'll get another blanket though.

L: Okay.

Me: Okay.

L: You're an alien, Mom. I'm not an alien, but you're an alien, so I must be an alien to you.

Me: I'm not an alien, I'm just your mom.

L: But this isn't my planet.

Me: What does your planet look like?

L: It's purple. Mountains.

Me: Mountains... does it have lakes or oceans?

L: Purple lakes, no oceans. Purple rivers, I guess. Purple water. Everything's purple.

Me: Sounds pretty.

L: Yeah, it's a good planet. Why aren't we on it? What planet are we on, Mom?

Me: We're on Earth.

L: Earth?

Me: Uh-huh.

L: Oh.

Me: What's your planet called?

L: I don't know. Are you sure?

Me: Yeah.

L: That we're on Earth?

Me: Yep. It's the best one.

L: Okay, yeah, okay.

L: I still want to go home to my planet. It's so purple and pretty.

Me: You'll be there soon.

L: I miss my people. They're not really people, but I miss them.

Me: I bet they're really nice people.

L: It's us and the government.

Me: Is it a good government?

L: Oh yeah, it's so much better than the ones on Earth cuz we, we figure stuff out. You guys are idiots.

Me: You get stuff done?

L: Yeah. You're a weird specienese. Specienese?

Me: That's a weird word. L: Specienese, no... Me: Specienese?

L: Yeah.

Me: I like that word.

L: Yeah, it's true words, scientific. It's a word that I learned... our education system is better than yours too. I learned that in school.

Me: What other stuff do you learn?

L: We learn intergalactic languages.

Me: Wow, that's amazing!

L: In school! Intergalactic! Do you understand what that means? There's been zero world wars on our planet, and this planet has existed for longer than Earth itself.

Me: It sounds amazing.

L: Zero world wars; zero. You know why? Cuz we're smart.

Me: Yeah, you are.

L: We're smarter than you people. No offense, but everyone on Earth are idiots.

Me: You guys must be really smart.

L: We are.

Me: I can tell.

L: Because we spend a lot of alone time. On weekends I like to spend a lot of alone time, hiking up the purple mountains. Wait... do you have any pants for me yet?

September 24, 2015, sometime after midnight (age 12)

The dreaded text: *Mom, can you come in?*

L sat on her bed, a somber look on her face.

"I'm so sorry, Mom, I'm so sorry," she said. "It spread to my right leg."

I was speechless. All L could do was apologize to me, because even in her pain, she was focused on protecting me. We both knew what this meant. The look in our eyes could always tell a complete story. Over the years there were many things between us that were not spoken, but they were never left unsaid. They were communicated with perfect clarity through a knowing look, a kiss on the forehead, a squeeze of a hand. In this moment, we knew she would be confined to a wheelchair. Her world, which had already shrunk so much, just became smaller. She literally couldn't get out of bed, and in the middle of the night, with no wheelchair in the house, we were stuck.

I disassembled her scooter which was downstairs, and carried it up to her room, piece by piece, where I reassembled it so that at least she could scoot to the bathroom. Her anxiety was through the roof, and she was bordering on having a panic attack. I gave her some of the emergency Valium, knowing it would not help the pain but hoping that it would help her sleep, so that I could cry in private and figure out what to do.

My dad came over in the middle of the night to comfort me. He stroked my hair as I drifted into a fitful sleep on the couch for an hour or two. Jaz stayed home from school that day. She has an incredibly loving heart and knew she just wanted to be home, needed to be home. As soon as stores opened, my dad went out and got a wheelchair for L. I called Dr. Lubenow. L was scheduled for another ketamine treatment the following week, and he was hoping that since the treatment was so close to when the pain had spread, that it would at least be able to knock it out of her right leg.

I carried L downstairs to a guest bedroom and helped her set up shop there so that at least she would have the freedom to wheel into the kitchen and get herself food without needing help. I was hoping her relocation to the downstairs bedroom would be short-lived.

September 29–October 29, 2015 (age 12)

More ketamine. They kept increasing the dosage. No results. Each time, as L woke up, she would talk about how she didn't want to be a burden to me, how she was so sorry and felt so guilty. I'd reassure her that she wasn't a burden, and the doctors would comment on her wisdom and compassion. At one point, between profuse apologies, she launched into a stand-up (well, a lying-down) comedy routine in which she played the character of our nosy, well-intentioned neighbor who was always offering us lasagna. She had the resident doubled over in laughter, telling me that he wasn't sure if he should laugh or cry listening to her.

Each day they gave her a few hundred more milligrams of ketamine, hoping for the breakthrough. On her final day, when they gave her so much that she couldn't wake up—and when she finally did, she had so much tightness in her chest and trouble breathing that I worried she was having a heart attack— we concluded that ketamine was not going to work for her.

November–December 2015 (age 13)

As L turned 13, the only remaining option was a surgical procedure to implant a spinal cord stimulator. The idea is that they place leads in the spinal cord that send electrical impulses to block the pain. At best, they reduce the pain by 50 percent, which is then hopefully enough to allow the patient to reengage in physical therapy for a more complete resolution. The risk is that any surgery can trigger a spread of the pain, plus there are people messing with your spinal cord. Seeing no other choice, we agreed to give it a try. The doctors first do a trial to see if it works; if it does, they schedule the surgery for permanent implantation.

Her trial was a few days before Thanksgiving. I waited anxiously to see her in the recovery room, to see if it brought her any pain relief. When I walked into recovery, I saw her awake with her legs resting on the bed. It was one of the more beautiful sights I had seen. The pain was still intense, she would tell me, but she could at least put her legs down. The permanent stimulator was placed on December 15 without complication. Our hope was that she would, over time, be able to increase her tolerance to touch and pressure so that she could get back on her feet. She came home and put on her first pair of pants, fuzzy *Little Mermaid* pajama pants, which she was able to tolerate for 10 minutes. Over many months, she was able to increase this until she could wear pants all day. In our world, this was a major accomplishment.

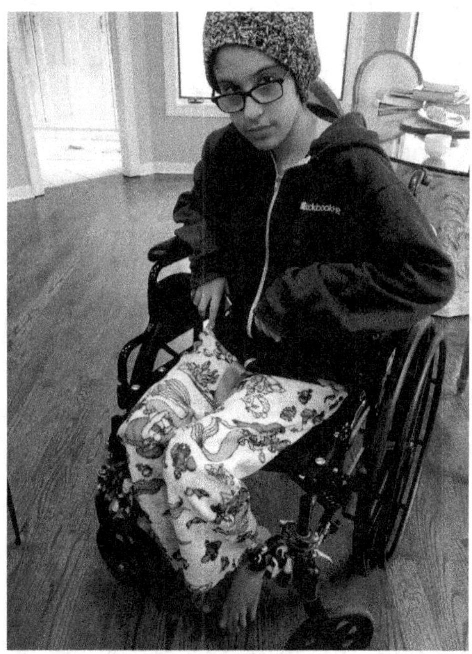

L wearing pants for the first time in 6 months, after her spinal cord stimulator was placed. Dec. 2015, age 13.

In the time following the surgery, we were hopeful that the slow progress would be steady and we would be on the path to recovery. It had been eight months at this point. Perhaps by summer she could be on her feet a little and, more importantly, her pain would decrease.

L worked hard—really hard. She wanted to get better more than anything. She pushed herself. And she also knew a truth the rest of us didn't (or wouldn't) allow ourselves to know.

L was a gifted writer—she always had been. She found that perhaps the best outlet for the pain, both physical and mental, was to write about it. She was determined to get published. She knew she had important things to say, that through her words she could elicit deep, powerful emotions in others, and she could speak her deepest truths.

"One day, Momma, when I am all better, you can read what I wrote. But not now, not while I'm sick. It would be too hard for you," she would say.

During the summer of 2018, after she passed, as I pored over every word she had written, I realized something I should have known all along. L knew everything. She knew from the very beginning that there would be no remission for her, that she would never get better. I finally began to see how little we'd understood, how she had been carrying the pain of all of our desperation, all of our wishing, all of our hope, all of our denial—and how profoundly and devastatingly lonely that was for her.

The poems, journal entries, and random thoughts of hers that I've reproduced here are printed exactly as she wrote them. I did not correct spelling, edit, capitalize letters, or add punctuation. There is a power in reading her original words, raw and unedited. Her use of grammar, or lack thereof, a direct reflection of her state of being.

Untitled
L Grey
November 15, 2015 (age 13)

its an inexplicable part of my existence that i am condemned to spend every day up to the eyes in pain. every waking minute in agony. fighting an unrecognized war, an unappreciated truth. with no audience to see my fight, no one to see my triumph, and no one to see my inevitable defeat. and even though some people care, they do not and will never understand that war. and that is why i will push them away. people will imagine idealized versions of my reality. it doesn't matter that its wrong. i have to believe its random, because if it's not, god is unimaginably cruel.

Fear
L Grey
November 21, 2015 (age 13)

The pain isn't going to break me. The hunting will.
I can't do this anymore. Look for the miracle answer. It's not there.
Everybody thinks they have it but the truth is, nobody does. call it
acceptance, call it living life, call it giving up.
I won't waste my life fighting a war I will lose.

Future?
L Grey
November 23, 2015 (age 13)

I'm scared for the future, because I know what it will entail.
I will graduate in pain.
Go to college in agony.
While peers tremble over lovers and grades,
I will be here, toiling day in and day out just to keep my head above water.
Trying not to drown in pain.
Everything I do, I do in pain.
I'll spend my life alone, pushing people away, because it's too tiring to
lie about.

Suffer:
L Grey
November 23, 2015 (age 13)

I've suffered enough. I don't want to die, but god, I don't care if I live

Entry 4:
L Grey
November 24, 2015 (age 13)

A life in solitude, toiling in
anonymity war tales untold but
surely felt caring ears completely
baffled uniquely alone, in a way
never known
I will push away those who care, because the pain of them not understanding while believing that they do, does more damage than loneliness ever could

Medicine:
L Grey
December 4, 2015 (age 13)

the thing is, i have looked harder for an answer than anybody who
has criticized me. Just because there isn't one, doesn't mean i haven't
worked my ass off to find it.
I will always be bitter that because of a few doctors idiocy and egos,
some family and friends alike doubted me, thought I was not trying
hard enough, or at all. thought i didn't want to get better. I will be bitter
that i was blamed for this, accused of being lazy, or too stubborn.
The painfully unfortunate truth is, that things happen for no reason sometimes. people with severed spines walk, people with acid in their eyes see,
these times when medical fact is baffled. I am blessed to be on the
opposite end of that spectrum, I did everything, EVERYTHING, right. but i
will be in pain the rest of my life. I will be crippled and in pain for the rest
of my life and I fucking shouldn't be. I will be at the hand of others'

*desperation, desperation to cure pain. i will live my life in denial,
because everybody else will live in denial. Where medicine meets art,
triumph meets tragedy. and i, i meet my fate.*

Stupid Ideas Part 2:
L Grey
December 11, 2015 (age 13)

*obsessive curiosity is my biggest virtue and worst vice
i cope by researching things
i haven't just seen hell, I've lived it
some of us don't have the luxury of not knowing agony
its not that i love being alone, its just that i don't have another choice. i
have people who care, but i don't have people who understand
this isn't the kind of pain that makes you stronger. It's not the kind that
you can learn from, it's the kind that makes you want to die.
this pain is every shred of happiness and youth burning to death.
I'm not an ass, I'm in pain.*

Hope
L Grey
December 2015 (age 13)

*"What's the most dangerous thing you have ever done?"
"Had hope, when every rational bone in my body knew otherwise. Hope is
devastating. It is denial and desperation mixed with fear and despair hid-
ing behind a fractured mask of innocent positivity. But it's never just that.
It's always dangerous games of denial. We all play them.
We have all lost a battle against groundless hope.
Had it take over. Rule us. Made us feel happy. Warm to the future, it's
reminded us that the future has something better in store. That it will be ok.
But then it's not. It's not ok. It's not better. Nothing changes.
And while you try to rekindle the fractured pieces of your soul, hope
laughs in a corner, singing a haunting melody-
Told you so..."*

L was thoughtful, she was complex, and she was suffering immeasurably. Her writing reflects the intricacies of her mind. Deep pain, bitterness, anger, loneliness, and soul-searching, all punctuated by moments of acerbic humor.

Hemingway contest ideas:
L Grey
November 6, 2015 (6 days shy of 13)

1; dying is painless, living kills you.

2; I've always been in pain, always screaming

3; what's it like? happiness, i mean.

4; that's oxymoronic, actually, just moronic

5; i should not be this strong

6; wasn't even love that broke me

8; the point is to find one

9; the greatest people are never understood

10; music reminds me I'm not alone

11; body hates me, thoughts segregate me

12; i miss the memories, not you

13; cold because my rage is not

14; i was powerless, on the ground

15; ernest hemingway: I'm ripping him off

16; hello, god? cut it out already

17; my cat wrote this one. meow

18; meow meow meow meow meow meow

19; my cat is a fucking artist

20; yes, i do my own stunts

21; this ones not artistic at all

22; "hey have you tried doing-" "yes"

23; pushing through shit is my specialty

24; *great people aren't well adjusted*

25; *easy is just a fucking lie*

26; *that night, the monster killed me*

27; *meant to make life, ended mine*

28; *she thought the shame was hers*

29; *people never get what they deserve, ever*

30; *only idiots and mothers make plans*

31; *i know how to make pain art*

32; *sorry, i didn't mean to die*

33; *virginity should never be stolen, ever*

34; *i lost my way, and mind*

35; *I'm not a tragedy, I'm powerful*

36; *hey, trust me, not the mirror*

37; *shut up and count your blessings*

38; *trust me, your legs look fine*

40; *some people don't get a childhood*

41; *ignorant towards others pain, not mine*

42; *not a victim, not a cripple.*

43; *labels are for food, not me*

44; *don't just let me get away with it*

45; *my truth traps me, labels me*

46; *my shrink testified- for the defense*

47; *sorry you saw me that way*

50; *i hate to see you sad, momma*

51; *i know melancholy so damn well*

52; *they read my diary in court*

53; *its ok, everybody always doubts me*

55; *I'll never wear out shoes again*

57; sick kid, most experienced med student

58; some people can't wear out shoes

60; my problems include stairs and stares

61; there's no more room for empathy

62; and i fell in love with melancholy

63; made to be cold and bitter

65; I'm sorry the pain is familiar

66; I'm terrified that I'll be average

67; pain didn't change me, you did

68; not a journey, this is hell

69; i like breaking rules

70; when's my funeral asked the president

71; so, what made YOU a cynic?

72; i trust myself, and that's it

73; what went wrong, what went wrong?

74; what the hell have i become?

75; all I do, i do in pain

76; and I'm to live in agony

77; i know agony all too well

78; Does it ever end? Does it?

79; Why do you have guns, officers?

80; "Radio Silence, good plan, Mr. president

81; "Blind Seer". Need i say more?

90; What if my legacy is suicide?

91; "They won't believe you" he taunted

92; "What got stolen, Miss?" "My virginity"

93; For Sale: Pretty Girl. Used nightly.

94; I am the god I fear

2016 (age 13)

On the surface it looked like things might be stabilizing. L's pain was not getting better, but she was so good at hiding it that most people could be around her and assume she was okay, or at least okay enough. Her pain wasn't decreasing, but she was slowly able to increase her tolerance to touch. She began wearing pants all day long, and when she could muster the energy, she was able to leave the house for brief excursions. We'd often grab a peanut-butter frozen yogurt and drive down Sheridan Road, getting lost in the beauty of the trees as L would go on one of her notorious "rants" about the social injustices of the world.

Early in 2016, L seemed to have a glimmer of hope about her future. "When I'm better, I want to get a tattoo of a flame on my left ankle… ya know, to remember. You down with that? Do you feel me?" "I'm down with that. I feel you."

Bucket List:
L Grey
January 2016 (age 13)

-Go to Japan

-Extreme long boarding down a steep hill in a tiny European town (90mph)

-Create a Eastern European Chess website called Czech Mate

-Be published in a well-known journal

-Get black stiletto nails

-Go to Tanzania

-Go to Iceland

-Get really lost and be the one who leads the group to safety

-Fly in somebody's private jet

-Have coffee with a killer (and not be killed)

-Have a sit-com level nice apartment

-Have a German Shepard

-Wear combat boots to a job interview, and get the job

-Internationally known

-Win a prize (Pulitzer, Oscar, Nobel, it all works)

-Pull off an incredibly elaborate prank

-Find my person. The Jane to my Daria, Patrick to my SpongeBob, Watson to my Sherlock, Wilson to my House. Be truly understood and not alone.

-Skydiving

-Scuba diving

-Finish a chapstick without losing or destroying it

-Be less inclined to justify myself while also being less of an ass-wipe

-Start a flash mob

-Learn to play an instrument

-Become fluent in another language. Preferably two.

-Be anything but average. Always bold, always pushing boundaries.

-Be the best "go to guy" in whatever it is I do

-Say "I made it" with all the truth in the world

-Publish a book by 25

-Wear out a pair of shoes again

-Be ok if I don't wear out a pair of shoes again

-Befriend an A-list celeb

She also became increasingly aware that there was more going on with her, physically, than the CRPS.

"Ever heard of Ehlers-Danlos Syndrome?" she asked me one day.

"No," I said. "What is it?"

"It's a connective tissue disorder, and I'm pretty sure I have it. There are several types, but the type I think I have is the hypermobility type. It's characterized by excessive joint hypermobility, slow wound healing, and easy scarring. One of the main ways doctors diagnose it is by having people bend their thumbs, like this." She contorted her thumb backward so that it was touching the back of her hand. "Your thumb doesn't do that, right Mom?" "No," I said, "it definitely doesn't. What made you look into it? Are you having symptoms beyond the CRPS?" I asked her the kind of questions I would later ask her doctors, because I knew she had researched it excessively at this point.

"I've been having some joint pain, so I started researching," she told me. "It's genetic, there isn't really a cure, and it usually gets progressively worse as people get older. Joints can start to dislocate all the time, it can cause problems breathing, all kinds of fucked-up shit. There is a high comorbidity with CRPS, but no one is quite sure why. I'm thinking it's why I used to twist my ankles all the time, and why my swim coaches yelled at me for hyperextending my elbows and shoulders."

"How much joint pain do you have? And why didn't you tell me sooner?" "It kind of crept up on me, and I didn't want to worry you. My joints hurt all the time, but it's minor in comparison to the CRPS pain. So, anyway, yeah, I thought it was time for you to know. You can go now; I want to be alone. Just wanted to give you a heads up."

I started researching EDS and specialists who could treat it. Everything L told me was correct. It could vary significantly in terms of how debilitating it was, and there was no cure, only management. The geneticist in Chicago who specialized in it had a two-year waiting list. I put my name on the list and asked the nurses to call me if anything opened up sooner. I asked Dr. Lubenow about it, and he said our primary goal needed to be getting the CRPS under control. Everything else would have to wait.

Her progress, if we could call it that, was agonizingly slow, and she and I both continued our research into any and every potential treatment that showed promise. We discovered there were some doctors who were experimenting with low-dose naltrexone to combat the pain. In high doses, naltrexone is given to people who have overdosed on opiates. Because CRPS creates physiological changes in the brain similar to those found with opiate use, some cutting-edge doctors discovered that low doses of naltrexone can begin to reverse the course of CRPS. None of these doctors were in Chicago, but a colleague of mine gave me the name of Dr. Gary Kaplan, based in Washington, DC. He was a prominent pain doctor who was having success with naltrexone. I was able to get L an appointment in March of 2016.

Unsure of whether L would be able to fly (navigating air travel with a wheelchair was daunting, and I was not sure if changes in air pressure would exacerbate her pain), we drove to DC and visited Dr. Gary. He was extraordinarily thorough. He spent three hours with her that first day, getting an in-depth history of everything she had been through. He understood how ravaging this disease was, and he was the first one to connect her migraines, which had been increasing in frequency and intensity since the CRPS began, to the fire in her legs. He looked at her illness systemically and explained to us that all of her pain was part of the same constellation of issues. L's body was not able to regulate pain. It never had been. The slightest insult to her body would trigger a pain cycle that her body was not able to bring back down. He explained that she was likely missing an enzyme that helped her body rid itself of toxins. This build-up was essentially poison and was preventing traditional treatments from having any kind of impact (subsequent tests confirmed this, indicating extremely high levels of toxic molds and fungi in her body).

During a follow-up call, he explained that nothing was going to work until all of the toxins (molds, fungi, c. diff bacteria, etc.) were cleared. He told us this was a slow process that could take up to a year. There was a series of medications and supplements that L would need to gradually introduce, in specific sequences, in order to help her body process and clear toxins. He was happy to start the naltrexone but suggested we wait until she was a few months into the detox for it to have any real impact.

He also diagnosed her with EDS in about 30 seconds. He saw her contort her thumb (one of the standard medical tests) and watched her hyperextend her elbows.

"There is no doubt she has EDS," he told us.

"What do we do about it?"

"At the moment, not much. It is managed with physical therapy, by keeping the muscles surrounding the ligaments strong. Some of this L is already doing, particularly with her upper body exercises, but the rest requires her to be on her feet, and that's just not possible right now. There are other, more invasive treatments that involve multiple injections that stimulate the body to rebuild collagen and ligaments, but that is too high risk at the moment. Those kinds of aggressive injections could cause her CRPS to spread."

"Okay, but do we need to worry about the stress she is putting on her wrists, elbows, and shoulders? I mean, every time she transfers from her wheelchair to a bed or a couch, she is putting her full weight on her wrists to lift her body weight for the transfer. Do we have to worry about injury to those joints with that degree of stress placed on them?"

Dr. Gary paused. "Yes," he said. "We do need to worry about that. But we need to go one step at a time. We don't want the CRPS to spread further. That has to be our primary focus right now."

I had very mixed feelings. I was grateful for Dr. Gary's knowledge, thoroughness, honesty, and realistic view of what lay ahead of us. And I was sickened that here we were, almost a year in, and we were looking at another year, at least, before there was any meaningful relief.

If my feelings were mixed, L's were abundantly clear. She was dejected at the thought of yet another lengthy and uncertain course of treatment. She had gone with the hope of getting a prescription for naltrexone, hoping she could take medicine that would make her better, and that was that. She had wheeled out staring down one more never-ending process that held no guarantee.

Dr. Gary and his nurses would become part of our family over the next two-plus years. While L balked at first, she came to appreciate just how knowledgeable he was about the multiple wars being waged in her body, and just how committed he was to her care. He never bull-shitted us. He told us when he had answers and when he didn't. He told us when he could explain what was going on with her, and when he was as stumped as we were. During her last few months, I would talk to his office daily. And the tears they all shed when learning of her death were the tears that come from having tried *so hard* to save someone who, in the end, could not be saved.

By late spring of 2016, we had established some kind of rhythm. L was taking an extraordinary number of supplements and prescription drugs to try to detoxify her body, calm her nervous system, and reduce her pain. The only area in which we could see a notable difference was in her migraines. The migraines that had once come on every three weeks, keeping L in a pitch dark room and unable to speak, eat, write, or listen to music for three days at a stretch, had reduced in frequency and duration. They now popped up about every three to four months and would last about two days. In our world, this was a big win. The fire in her legs, however, continued to rage.

L was homeschooled at this point; she had been since her illness began. She would Skype in to her classes, and her math teacher, Ms. K, would come over each week under the guise of teaching L math, but really to be a lifeline. Their banter was salty, sarcastic, and brilliant. I loved coming home and seeing the two of them at the kitchen table. Whether they were engaged in intense debate or violent agreement, L's passion, which had always been a part of her but was often buried under so many layers of pain, shone bright and pure.

Ms. K became one of several lifelines for L. Her therapist, Sharon, would come to the house for their sessions, often with a frozen yogurt or a Starbucks in hand for L. Ultimately, she introduced L to Agatha who would become one of her closest friends throughout her illness. Her physical therapist, Melissa, would also come to the house. She knew exactly how much to push L, and she never assumed that she understood the full extent of L's pain. L trusted her. With Melissa she could push herself to the edge, and she could say "uncle" when she had had enough.

At some point, I installed a stairlift in the house. It was clear that L was not going to be out of her wheelchair anytime soon. The lift allowed her to move back into her room upstairs, where she felt more comfortable. With the lift, she could go up and down the stairs independently. We had also switched pediatricians, and L was now in the primary care of Jessica, a doctor who did not doubt L and knew that L was here to teach her as much as she was here to provide medical care to L. She appreciated L, respected her, and was impressed by her humor, attitude, courage, and grace. Perhaps most important was that she trusted L. She knew that L understood what was going on in her body better than anyone else could. She took her cues from L and viewed her role as being in service of L's well-being.

So, we had our routine, and it became our normal. I could go through the days with an illusion that things were bearable, willing the nagging voice in my head that threatened to tell me otherwise to quiet itself.

One of the many paradoxes of L was that she could maintain a certain duality. She carefully walked the line of doing her best to live in the moment, to strive for a better future, and coming to grips with the grim reality that lay ahead. She gave her all to getting better. She poured her heart out to Sharon, working through the trauma of the sexual abuse, the agony of being at the mercy of a legal system that failed her time and time again, the fear of the pain itself, the reality of coming to grips with being disabled, and her growing frustration over not being believed by certain people. She worked hard in physical therapy with Melissa. She followed Dr. Gary's protocol (except for the diet; L ate like a three-year-old). She made the wallpaper on her phone her medical ID so that if something were to happen while she was out of the house, people would know what to do and she would be safe.

She would find moments of pleasure, sometimes in something as simple as a good donut. She would find moments of humor with me, with her sister, with her teachers, and mostly with her friends. She read and she wrote. A lot. She taught herself to read music, to play the keyboard, and to read and speak Hebrew. She studied history and art, sociology and anthropology, quantum physics and biology. She was determined to use her mind. She talked about when she would be able to swim and ride her bike again, where she wanted to travel (Iceland and Japan topped the list), where she wanted to go to college, the quiet life with her wife and goats that she envisioned for herself. And throughout it all, she maintained a deep, solitary knowing that she would not be cured; that eventually, when she had endured all she could endure, the only way to end the pain would be to leave her expiring body behind. She hid this knowing in the same masterful way that she hid the full extent of her physical pain. Only in her writing could she describe what was indescribable —the pain itself, and the isolation of being alone in what she knew. During the spring of 2016, her words flowed freely.

Abyss Refill
L Grey
April 27, 2016 (age 13)

With pen in hand, I fight as I try desperately to write out the misery.
But it comes back, filling me from bottom up.
Like a force out of my power keeps getting free refills on this bottomless abyss.

Forfeit
L Grey
April 27, 2016 (age 13)

Naive Child, quitting now isn't rebelling, it's letting me win the game.

At Least They Knew They Were Alone
L Grey
May 15, 2016 (age 13)

Brilliant men go down in history as aliens,
but me- nobody knows of my isolation.
Assumptions and doubt included, being isolated with nobody aware of your departure from the real world is perhaps the worst form of hell there is. Lying to myself all I want, it's not that I care about others deluded opinions of me, I crave acknowledgment for my insatiable loneliness. Beethoven, Hemingway, Van Gogh and Picasso all went down in history as ingenious freaks. Their pain was noted, and people accepted that it was a pain they could never and would never know for themselves. They accept that these men would be condemned to an existence they would personally never understand. They accepted that, and they accepted their contributions to society, even if they were all enigmatic. I wish for my loneliness to be noted and appreciated, instead of having people try to fathom my life. I wish that instead of unsolicited advice from people that have never and will never know my anguish, that they could just accept that I am an enigma, and that they won't ever know my life, even if they are able to enjoy my writing.

There is nothing more agonizing and lonely than being alone and not one person in the whole world knowing that you are alone and in pain. Having them hold you to standards unreachable because they are blind to your suffering. Having them always doubt your claim of distress and a solitary life without any of the understanding that they will never understand. It's not that I wish for myself pity or even understanding, I just wish that people knew and would accept that they didn't understand me and that I am and always have been alone, and that that fact in and of itself is ok with me, if only it was common knowledge.

Stop trying to change me, to fix me, or to understand me. I know you think you understand me, even that you understand me and know me better then I know my own self. Go ahead, attribute this to teenage angst, but just remember that, when writing my legacy.

Deleted Draft
L Grey
May 16, 2016 (age 13)

Pain is too weak a word to explain this. I am on fire. Sledge hammers shatter charred bones. Muscles are squeezed in a vice. Thousands of pointed swords relentlessly stab me. I am all too aware of my erratic pulse. I cannot bear it, but somehow I do.

At night, as my daytime facade crumbles, exhaustion overcomes me, but getting so much as 2 or 3 hours of sleep is a luxury. I get dizzy and gasp for air. This isn't a nightmare I can simply wake up from in the morning, this is life. I panic.

What do I do? What can I do? There is hardly anything more terrifying than the knowledge that 24/7, everyday and every night will be like this, and nobody can change that. I am nauseous. I feel like I'm going to faint. If I could scream, I would, but instead I breathe through gritted teeth. I don't remember what it was like a year ago, when I wasn't in agony. I am so incredibly overwhelmed by the fact that I am unable to impart the knowledge of my existence onto anybody. We are the only people who know what it is like to physically be us, everyone is trapped inside their own body, but all the words in the world cannot convey the burden of being stuck in mine.

Don't Lecture
L Grey
May 17, 2016 (age 13)

don't lecture me about the war, you didn't fight in it

Migraines
L Grey
May 21, 2016 (age 13)

My dear, you kiss me with the force of breaking waves
Clouding vision like a sandstorm reign
Laying sullied top to bottom
You fend for your prestige
The cavalry has ravaged this land
Watch forests retaliate with new growth
Your kiss though halts the war
Escape daunts with its dilemma
When pondering strategy is undoable
Hostile to thoughts, chained to a dark room
Isolated from even myself

Requiem for me
L Grey
May 21, 2016 (age 13)

Tonight, I sing a silent requiem for the self I lost along the way, The parts that died on the journey coming here. Tonight, I shed a tear for a who I used to be

(I can't) Write this away
L Grey
May 27, 2016 (age 13)

No words can explain this.
In all the similes and metaphors,
I don't know how to convey my body.
I can write away the rotting sadness,
Or searing rage,
But how do I make somebody know my pain?
How do I transfer anguish that's not human?
It's not a question of verse or prose; I simply cannot do it
I can write away the isolation
I can write away the frustration,
But I cannot write this away

I Write
L Grey
May 27, 2016 (age 13)

I write because it hurts.
I write to soothe the pain.
I do it to become somebody who isn't me, in a world that isn't mine.
I write so the way I lived and the things I thought don't die with me.
I write to express and repress
I do it to shape the future and mend the past.
I write because if I didn't, I'd be empty.
I write so I can be immortal
I write because a blank page will always understand me.

L knew that our souls were interconnected, her suffering almost indistinguishable from mine. She knew that, in different ways, her illness was quietly and slowly killing both of us.

Slain/fates
L Grey
April 27, 2016 (age 13)

You were numb, I am burning. together, we were slain.

As I opened each file, read all of her words, it was clear that May 29, 2016, was a particularly tumultuous day for her. On that day she was able to capture the physical pain, the abuse, the mental anguish, and the façade we were all trying desperately to maintain. I wish I could remember what was going on that day, but my guess is that, on the surface, it was a "regular" day in this strange, surreal universe we found ourselves in.

I Ran Once
L Grey
May 29, 2016 (age 13)

I escaped from the tongue that licked my cheeks
now show me to run from the flames that lick my feet
I wriggled free from bayonet words but how
do I kill the machine guns at my knees
I ran from a dungeon and fumbled through years
teach me how to eat the nails I step on

At Night
L Grey
May 29, 2016 (age 13)

I am swimming through concrete and nobody sees.
At night I can barely breathe because the rise and fall of ribs is a gro-
tesque form of torture. Each 'up' sending electric currents and the
'downs' a chainsaw skinning me.
I almost can't see, like my brain is so overwhelmed with the job of feel-
ing it eats up light

After a performance of health for 18 hour days I don't scream. If I could I would but screaming takes energy I don't have. Instead I lay as silently still as I can, taking in as few breaths as possible in the form of gasp or groan or a cry out to the ceiling.

My mother offers to sit with me, but I don't let her. My agony is my secret. In the morning my hands hurt from the fists they held all night and my eyes sag from the lack of sleep

Throughout the day I trudge over mountains to keep up with myself I leave my life to go to bed and yell bloody hell into a pillow, because I am allergic to morphine, so anger is all I have to kill the pain.

And sometimes it was her brevity that told the most poignant story. The combination of this title, and the four words that follow, speak volumes.

Mom
L Grey
May 29, 2016 (age 13)

pretend, pretend for me

And, of course, these three words.

My Mind
L Grey
May 29, 2016 (age 13)

Let

Me

Go

Throughout all of it, she remained intensely protective of me. It is clear that over the years she would contemplate taking her life by her own hand as a last resort to end the pain. May 29th was one of those days. And I have no doubt that she survived being burned alive for an additional two years beyond that day to protect me from the anguish of losing a child and to shield Jaz from the heartache of losing her sister. This was her last entry on May 29, 2016.

Goodbye, then

L Grey

May 29, 2016 (age 13)

Mom- I love you. Always will. You were the best thing in my life. I'll miss you every day. Be happy, for me. Please mommy, you deserve it. To inflict what I have inflicted on you is unforgivable. You were the light of my life. You are too damn good for this cesspool of a world. I know you want to, but don't kill yourself tonight. When you get there, send me a letter from the light, ok?

Jaz- I'm sorry. Live on. Live boldly. Live freely. Be happy. Never settle. You are inimitable. I love you, Angel.

Mom, Grazer is for you. He was a comfort for me, maybe he can do the same for you. Jaz, camera is for you. Let it capture all the joyful moments I know you will have.

Please take my glasses. Try to imagine what I saw every day.

Please cremate my useless body. Sprinkle me in Japan. I always wanted to go.

I didn't want to kill myself. I wanted to kill the pain. Unfortunately, the two are little lovebirds, always together- inseparable.

Goodnight.

But she had too much to say, too much to do, too many causes to which she would need to give voice, and she was too worried about us to succumb to the pain just yet. So, she soldiered on with words on her tongue that needed to find their way to print, and the reminder of what it would be like for a mother to lose a child as her beacon.

My Daughter Cut Her Hand
L Grey
May 17, 2016 (age 13)

One dusk last June my daughter played outside.
She climbed up trees and ran about and sat down on a swing.
Back and forth she swung all night
before she fell down to the ground.
Her hand was cut on a wooden beam,
but she didn't make a sound.
It burned and ached but she was silent when she came back to the house.
It bled through every bandage, but she did not make a sound.
She never told me of her cut,
Assuming I'd be mad.
One day I felt her head was warm and her body shook like fear
I saw that red hot hand of hers and asked her to explain
"I cut it on the swings that night"
was all she ever said
They gave her pills for the cut
And she took them everyday
They gave her pills for the infection
But it wouldn't go away
It made it from her hand to heart,
and it killed her that July.
Ravaged, broken, beaten down
Because she did didn't make a sound
My daughter died. Gone, forgotten
From just a cut upon her hand
My baby died, and now, somehow,
Alone, I must survive.

Perspectives
L Grey
June 6, 2016 (age 13)

I write poetry from the perspective of a grieving mother whenever I feel suicidal.

Her writing was an outlet for the pain but also a force, much like gravity. She knew she had the ability to capture with her words a depth of emotion and an authenticity that most people struggle to fully tap into. And she felt compelled to put her words on paper so that they did not die with her, so that somehow, some way, maybe her ability to describe the complexity of the human condition would help others on their own path. If protecting me was one of the reasons she endured what she did for so long, she was equally motivated by getting as much on paper as she possibly could. She was driven by the need to speak her truth, all of her truth, and to make it known to the world around her.

Manic Thoughts
L Grey
May 20, 2016 (age 13)

manic thoughts that don't let me sleep. I have to get them out or else they die. And who am I to play god with what thoughts get to live and which must die. Then, it takes me time to give a voice, to find the right eloquent words to suit each thought. But when I do, It's magic even when I am so tired I cannot keep my eyes open, so tired I am taking cat naps on my keyboard. so sick I can't get out of bed, and I have to be careful to only move my fingers on the keys, and not type too hard, because the pressure hurts, I still have to open up my laptop and write whatever poem or story or whatever i need to get out.
It's why I hate migraines so much. Because all I have to entertain me are my thoughts, but I cannot write anything. I cannot express my isolation on the island of pain. it's terrible and lonely.

TURN THIS OUTLINE INTO SOMETHING L THIS IS JUST FOR NOW CAUSE YOU ARE WORKING ON SOMETHING MORE DIRE. THIS IS LIKE NOTES L THAT YOU JUST HAD TO JOT DOWN WHILE DOING A DIF-FERENT PROJECT ENTIRELY. PLEASE COME BACK TO THIS FUTURE SELF.

Not Yet
L Grey
May 17, 2016 (age 13)

I've had friends who've died in battle from broken necks and wrists torn open
I've lost kin each day from this grisly, gory, crimson altercation
And it'd be deceit for me to say I haven't wished for abdication
But I cannot relinquish my role just yet
Departing now as a final act would tarnish all past toil
To leave me little known and never by my name
There's still a starving pang that I must feed
It's not a want but rather a violent need
If I go now I'll be soon forgotten, defined by one act I presented
But if I stay I have the time to imprint minds
So I can demand a space for me,
So in my absence nobody can replace me
Because I will not go another face
And I cannot leave so out of place
I have to make my mark, to show I fought in brawls a many, To show I
made my way even in thick density If leaving now is destiny,
Then a single act of cowardly retreat becomes the former me
I will not let one show of weakness embody my legacy
Even if it means clawing up with every cross I ever bore
With broken feet, outrunning time to brand a world that was never mine
A world that wasn't ready to see,
An area not meant for me
I will sculpt my sorrow into a powerful choir
To make sure the sound still lingers tomorrow
Average, alone, I will not go
Not yet. Not ever.

And, of course, there were just some perfectly crafted one-liners.

Blah
L Grey
September 8, 2016 (age 13)

poets are just those among us who can speak with enough grace to make their words palatable, and enough truth to make it hurt.

At the end of 2016, we got Evie, the cutest Cavalier King Charles spaniel imaginable. L was instantly in love. She was calmer with Evie by her side, and as the puppy weighed just four pounds, L was able to tolerate her being on her lap. A four-pound weight on her lap was an extraordinary accomplishment. L's smile busted through the pain as Evie nuzzled into her neck, and I went into 2017 feeling modestly hopeful.

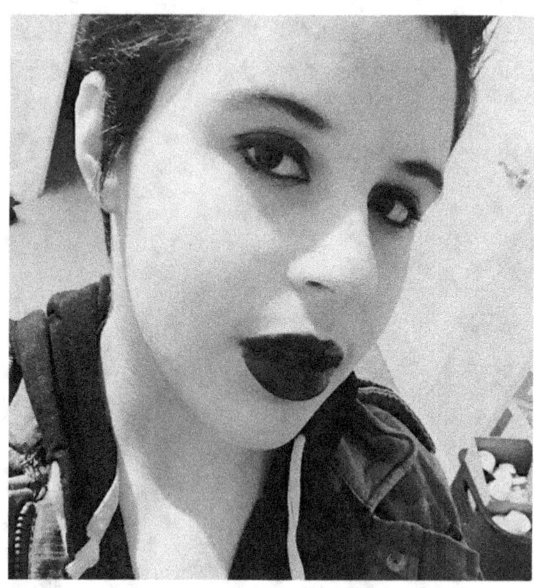

L, 2016, age 13.

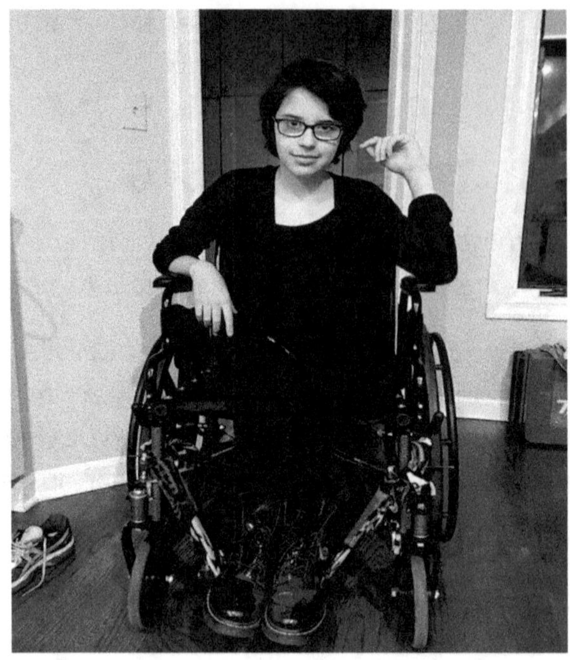

L wearing shoes for the first time since getting sick, 2016, age 13.

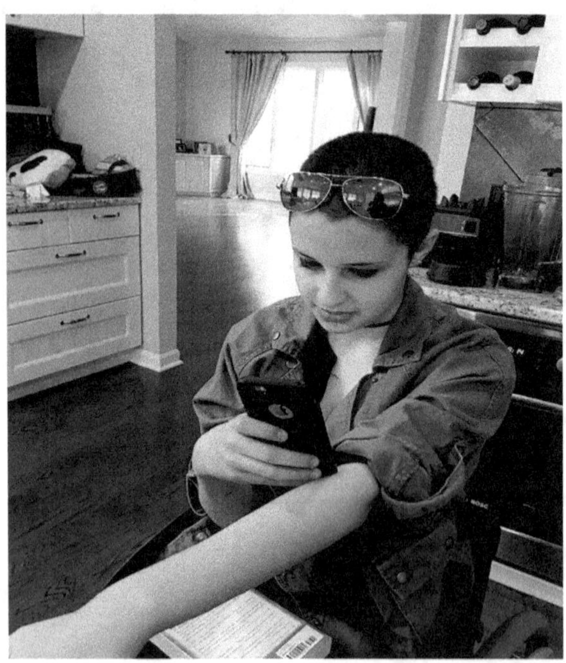

L, taking my breath away, 2016, age 13.

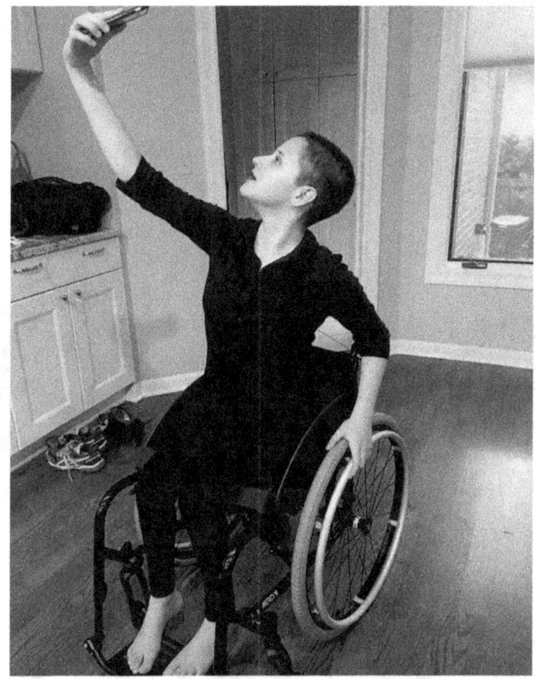

L, triumphant, 2016, age 13.

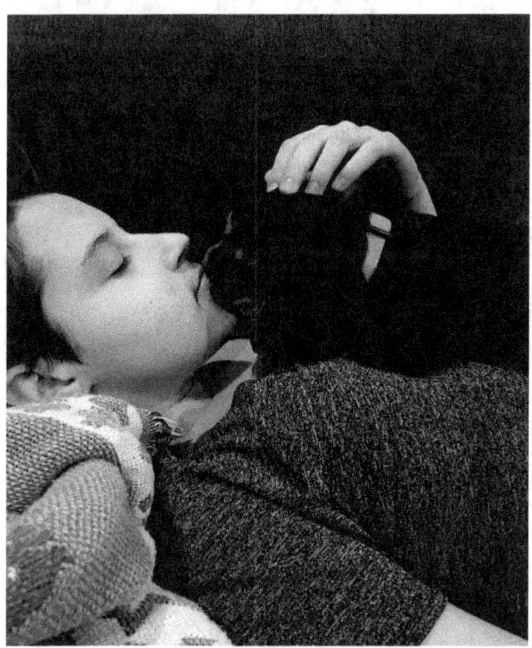

L and Evie, December 2016, age 14.

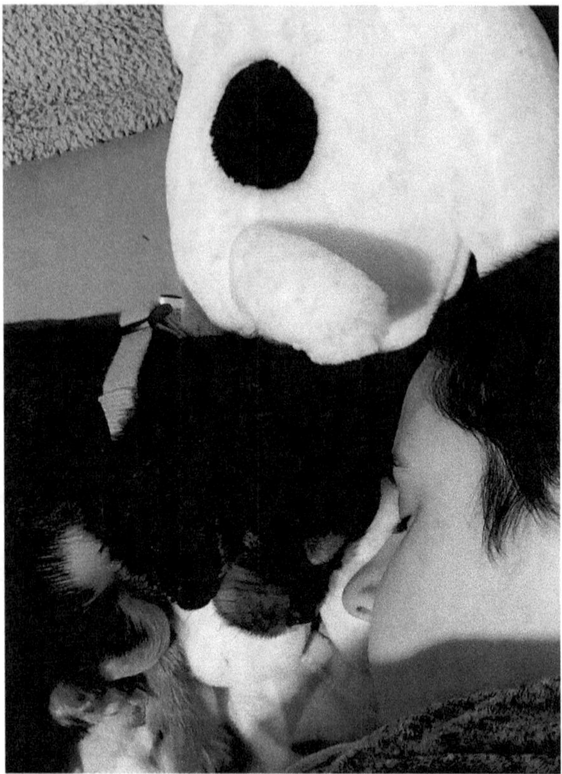

L and Evie, December 2016, age 14.

2017 (age 14)

Once you hit the two-year mark of CRPS, the prognosis is not good. The research shows that after two years, the odds of remission drop precipitously. The curse of L's curiosity was that she researched everything, and she knew more about this disease than most. There was no hiding the truth of what she was facing. She knew it, I knew it, and we knew that it was a shared understanding. It was one of the many things we didn't need to verbalize. We were both painfully aware of time marching on and how rapidly April 21, 2017, was approaching.

Nevertheless, L kept pushing. She followed Dr. Gary's regimen almost to the tee, with the exception of his recommendations on diet. He wanted her off any kind of inflammatory food, which meant no gluten, no sugar, no dairy. Intellectually, L was incredibly sophisticated. But when it came to her palate, she preferred pizza, fries, macaroni and cheese, and ice cream. Her eating habits were another one of the few childlike qualities of L, and she was intensely stubborn about changing them. "It is one of the few things that still brings me joy," she would plead with me. I understood that, I really did. But I also couldn't leave any potential stone unturned. So, we made a deal. We would eat "clean" together. No gluten, no dairy, no sugar for either of us. And we would do it for two months (per Dr. Gary's recommendation). If we saw no improvement in her symptoms, she could go back to eating what she liked.

Twice throughout the course of 2017 we would do this two-month "clean" diet. Neither time did it do anything to change her symptoms. Dr. Gary reluctantly agreed. If eating clean was not going to bring her any relief, then it was just cruel to deny her something that could make her smile. So, pizza, ramen noodles, and Starbuck's Frappuccinos were back in rotation. In retrospect, I am grateful they were. With a body that was failing her, at times a perfect bite of food was the only thing that could make the day seem bearable. Sometimes on weekends I'd make her Pillsbury cinnamon rolls, glopping extra icing on top as they came hot out of the oven. And I can honestly say, there were times when the bliss brought about by the sugary perfection transcended the pain, even if just for a microsecond. I'm grateful for that. Exceptionally grateful for that.

Aside from her transgressions in eating, L did everything her doctors instructed her to do. One of the more impressive things to me during this time was how gracefully she was able to come to terms with her disability. Reconciling that you may spend the rest of your life in a wheelchair is hard for an adult to fathom, let alone a 14-year-old. Yet she did more than fathom it. She came to accept it, to embrace it, to be open to the possibility that she may walk again, but to be content if she didn't. She was prepared to live her life in a wheelchair, and she figured out how it could be a full life. She looked that beast in the eye and wrestled it to the ground, and she didn't look back.

On Being Crippled, On Being Proud
L Grey
July 2017 (age 14)

We are not seen as human.
Our bodies are perceived as graveyards, as tragedies, as a terrifying what-if.
They are scrutinized from top to bottom.
They are specimens in a lab.
They are broken.
They are pity.
We are seen as unlovable. Unfuckable. Undesired. Unwanted.
Objectified and thrown away.
Fetishized.
We see our bodies- our lives- played out for laughs and tears on screen.
There is no dignity in being an oddity.
Privacy is not a luxury we have.
There are too many eyes.
Curious, unforgiving eyes.
We are gossip at a dinner party. Our stories are whispered as small talk
when they think we cannot hear.
Our stories are taken from us.
They try and fix us.
Our broken, beautiful, unfixable bodies.
And they don't ever succeed.
We try and wash off the words.
Wash off the pity.
Pray the steam will ease the pain.
Grieve for the identities we've lost. The identities we never had. We
welcome the new ones that were born.
We have been poster children and freak show attractions.
Prisoners and studies.
We have crawled our way to justice.
We have taken pride in the taboo. Reclaimed our lives.
Mastered the art of being broken.
So beautifully, perfectly, pridefully broken.

Every scar, every bruise, every useless muscle.
Until there is no more shame to wash away.

It was not the prospect of living her life disabled that terrified her. It was the prospect of living the rest of her life *burned at the stake* that did.

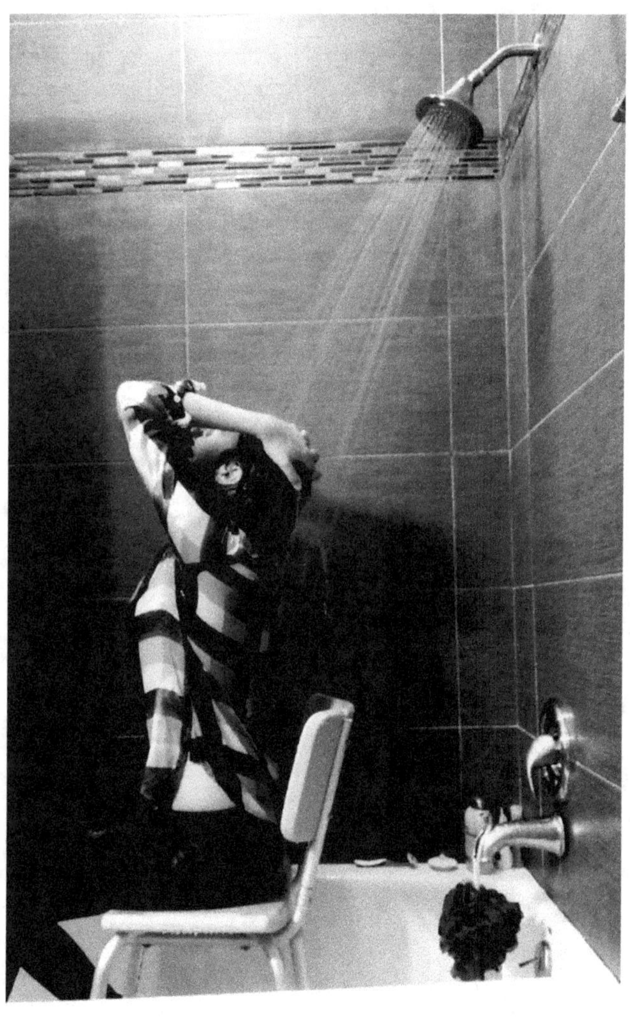

L, self-portrait found in her computer alongside
"On Being Crippled, on Being Proud," July 2017, age 14.

February 2017 (age 14)

The winter of 2017 was relatively stable in the makeshift world we were living in. There weren't any major breakthroughs, nor were there major setbacks, and through the pain there were always glimmers of L's humor. They came THROUGH in random moments as we were going about our day-today lives, and the best we could do was hold those moments for as long as time would allow. Here's one text exchange between the two of us from February 2017. I took a screenshot of it at the time because it made me laugh.

After her death, as I looked through everything on L's phone, I realized that she took a screen shot of it as well, both of us somehow driven to memorialize our laughter. Seeing her screenshot would be one of the many gifts L gave me, and one of the many ways she would communicate with me after she died. Looking through all of the photos on her phone, so many of which were taken in hospitals, documenting the progression of her illness, was an unbearable task. And in the moments when I could barely see through my tears, tucked in between photos of lesions and infections, she reminded me of who she really was, demanded I not drown in sorrow, and literally forced me to laugh out loud.

L: Can we have pizza for dinner?

Me: Pizza is good. Let me know where and what time L: Not in a Barnabys mood. Maybe La fornicate?

L: TYPI

L: TYPO. Damn you autocorrect

L: IL forno's

Me: I'm laughing so hard right now!!!

March 2017 (age 14)

Small milestones. We decided it was time to try to travel. I had been on a Southwest flight for business travel, and I saw that the aisle was wide enough for L's wheelchair, and if we got the bulkhead seat, L could wheel onto the plane, transfer to that seat, store her chair on the plane, and actually leave Chicago. L, Jaz, and I planned a trip to Arizona for spring break. The challenge would be that once seated, she would not be able to use the bathroom, and with a four-hour flight to Arizona, we would have to pray for no delays. We decided L wouldn't drink anything before the flight, and we would give her preventative migraine medication to ward off a dehydration-induced migraine. I was on edge, to say the least. I had no idea if the change in pressure would spike her pain, no idea what would happen if we were delayed. My only solace was that we were visiting a friend who was a physician at the Mayo Clinic, so I knew that once we landed we would at least have access to good medical care if we needed it.

The flight was remarkably, mercifully uneventful, and we spent five days in the Arizona sun. L spent the vast majority in the hotel room, reading and writing, but she would join us poolside for lunches and would go out for an occasional dinner. We discovered a pizza place that rivaled places we had eaten at in Italy, and for the first time in two years I was able to be on vacation with both of my girls. A world of possibilities seemed to open for us. With L being able to fly, we planned trips for that summer while Jaz was at camp. We would travel to the East Coast to visit some friends and to see Dr. Gary, and we would go back to Arizona. And we knew she would be able to return to Sanibel that Christmas, which somehow always felt more like home than our big house in Chicago.

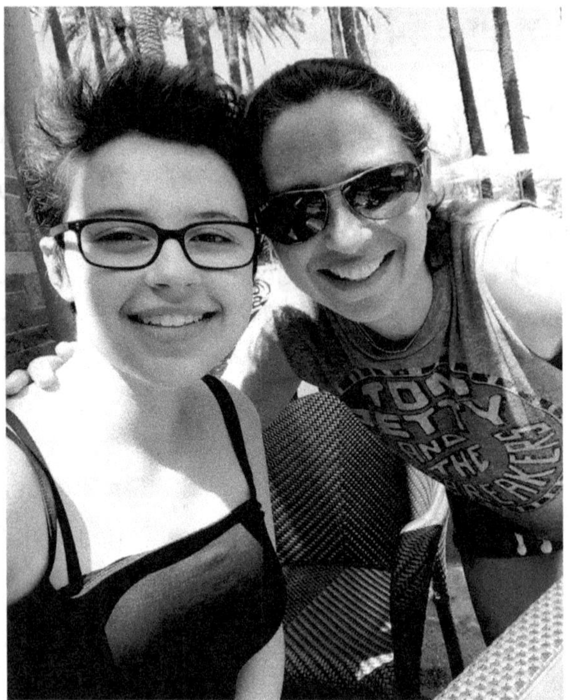

L and me in Arizona, March 2017, age 14.

April 21, 2017 (age 14)

L had an amazing ability to be a cheerleader and champion for Jaz, no matter what she was going through herself. So, when the day of Jaz's bat mitzvah arrived, no one was more proud of her than L. Jaz had worked hard, deciding on her own that she wanted to learn Hebrew and experience this Jewish rite of passage. It was time for celebration. For one night. It was also the two-year anniversary of the onset of L's illness. We knew what that meant. But L was a big sister at her core and was far too protective of Jaz to even mention it. She donned a tuxedo, did her hair and make-up, and looked more radiant than I had seen her look in years. She posed for pictures, mingled with relatives, celebrated Jaz and cheered her on with gusto, and gave a heartfelt speech, never flinching, never giving the slightest indication that she was on fire, never letting on that she knew what the day marked, never suggesting how frightened she was of the fate she was facing.

Bat Mitzvah Speech to Jaz

L Grey
April 21, 2017 (age 14)

Jaz, jaz, jaz

Mazel Tov. I know how much you've wanted this. I've seen all the hours and hours of work you've put in, and I know I speak for everybody in this room when I say we are all so incredibly proud of you. Congratulations, jaz. You've earned this.

In fact, you are one of the most hardworking, determined people I know. The amount of detail and effort you put into everything you do- whether it's your bat mitzvah or your homework or baking a cake- It's amazing to watch you work towards a goal, because when you want to achieve something, nothing on this earth can stop you. I hope you know that whatever it is you want, and whatever you need, I will always, always be here for you. I hope you know that, because I know that I could go to you with a problem, and you'd listen without judgement. I hope you know that I'd do anything for you, because I know you would for me.

I am amazed by you every day. You are always the most compassion-ate, loving person in the room, and everybody feels better when you're around. I admire your ability to see the best in everybody. We joke about the "jazzy love," but in truth, you really do have an almost inhuman capacity for loving and healing and niceness. You care so deeply for everybody you meet, your first priority is always the comfort of the person that you're with. You are selfless in a way the rest of us can only dream of being, and you stoically deal with any situation the comes your way.

It is an honor and a privilege to be your sister. I am so proud of you for everything you do, because you handle it with grace. You are stunningly beautiful, both inside and out. You are braver than you get credit for, but it doesn't go unnoticed. I am in awe of you every day.

You are the first friend I ever had, and the best one I ever will. I love you so much more than I can possibly express in a 2 minute speech.

Mazel Tov, Jaz.

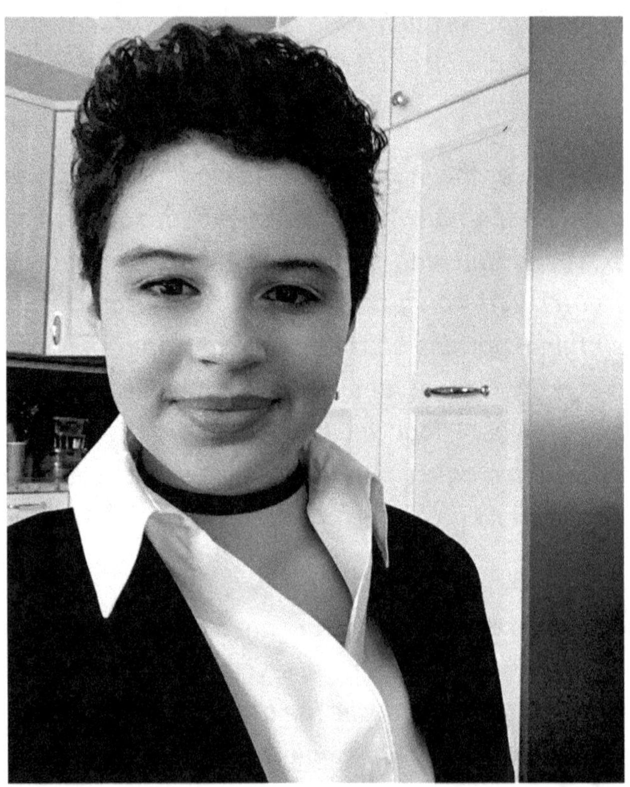

L at Jaz's bat mitzvah.

May 2017 (age 14)

Though her migraines were better controlled at this point, they would still come to visit periodically, robbing L of the ability to write. L wanted to document anything and everything that she was experiencing, and the frustration of not being able to do so was visceral. As soon as she could tolerate the light radiating from her computer screen, she would feverishly try to convey her thoughts from the preceding days. This stream-of consciousness account of migraine-induced dreams encapsulates so much of the complexity, sass, and beauty that was L.

Migraine Dreams
L Grey
May 2, 2017 (age 14)

Just to document my fucked up triptan induced dreams last night, now that the worst of the migraine has let up:

In no particular order, I was in some store, but it wasn't a store it was a hospital (but it was a store... with sick people and doctors) and I was with Siegel and her class for some assignment, wheelchair, Evie, schoolmates all present. Then some guy who was dying in a trauma bay exploded blood all over the place. Everything was covered in so much blood and it was suddenly Jaz's friends bat mitzvah in this bloody hospital store. I have Jack Cohens mom drive me home, but she only drove me to the train tracks and I walked home. Walked, even though Lori Gordon had to help her put my wheelchair in the car at the hospital-store-party. And then I was raiding Grey Swift's closet with mom to prove a point to Jaz. I'm kinda waking up at this point, sweaty and out of it but I go back to sleep.

Then I'm cutting power lines and flying across a battle field for a WWI assignment. Siegel is there again, and I'm flying over these suburban houses. I can't really remember but there was something about Harry Potter.

Then, the same empty battlefield and the woods behind it are filled with soldiers. Revolutionary War soldiers. But they're all actors from the show Turn but I don't know that, I think its actually c. 1776 because it IS in the dream. So I'm in the woods behind the battle field on a horse, and the guy riding the horse has really bad burn scars and is Matt Bomer (but i think he's some soldier) and I'm thinking in this 3rd person dream "I'm gay but this

guy is hot. I'd go straight for him." OK so we ride up to this little cottage and there's a woman there and she's "taking care of her son" and her son is Benedict Arnold, but not the actual Arnold the actor from Turn who plays Benedict Arnold.

Cut to the field, the woods on the horizon, tons of canons, but the cottage and the woman are there, right in the middle of the artillery. Inside the house is Arnold laying in bed all sweaty and feverish and dying, and I just know in the dream its cause he was shot but I know in my own dream that he's not the real Arnold, that this isn't historically accurate. But he's laying there, dying, but not really dying. And then I'm texting Wes asking what color pants Washington's army wore and he's in modern day times asking me "wtf" and then we start analyzing Pride and Prejudice while I'm just casually sitting by Benedict Arnold's bedside.

So then the same burned Matt Bomer horse guy shows up with 2 horses and takes me, the mom, and Arnold through the battle back to the woods (which is now a different woods) and Arnold is totally unconscious and just laying on this horse so I say "wait isn't he supposed to be bedridden?" because I think I'm the doctor in this dream and thats my best 18th century idea. lay in bed. So horse guy (who I'd still go straight for) says "no he is this counts because he's laying on the horse" and we go to this magical sun spot in this circular woods thing? and at this point I think "why is burned matt Bomer shirtless? why was Wes rude? what is this place? should I tell Washington that Arnold is a traitor?

And then we're back in this cottage and it's a month later and he's still in bed and there's still a battle.

I wake up and roll over (in real life) and that's the end of that clusterfuck.

I go back to sleep and have this hazy dream I don't really remember about a Russian plane crash and wedding? Idk it was a movie in the dream and it made me emotional in the dream.

So yeah I think migraines give me weird dreams because this is not the first time...

"Mom, you should know, I don't feel right. I mean duh, I have CRPS, and I know exactly what that pain feels like. But something else is going on. My whole body just doesn't feel right, beyond the CRPS. It's hard to explain, but everything is just off. I've been monitoring my heart rate and blood pressure, cuz, ya know, I'm me, so I do stuff like that. And I know my heart rate has been high, but sometimes I'm just sitting here in bed and it's like 170. And sometimes I feel like I'm going to pass out, and my blood pressure is like 90/60. There's other stuff too. I'm literally nauseous all the time. And I'm tired in a way I can't describe. It's hard for me to even open my computer sometimes. And I feel like the EDS is getting worse. Every joint in my body aches, and my shoulder has been dislocating a lot. Melissa taught me how to pop it back in, but, ya know, it's not fun." In addition to this, she had been randomly breaking out in hives triggered by no known allergen. Benadryl helped, but it certainly didn't explain what was going on.

Dr. Gary was not happy, nor was he surprised by her elevated heart rate, low blood pressure, and progression of joint pain. All are signs of progressing EDS. The best thing we could do at the moment was to keep her properly hydrated (turns out this is the most effective way of managing heart rate and blood pressure, and it is why the first thing hospitals do is start a saline drip), and do as much physical therapy as her body would allow.

Her other symptoms, he posited, could be a result of mast cell activation syndrome (MCAS). Mast cells have to do with the body's allergic responses, and in MCAS these cells fire on overdrive for no known reason. Little is known about it, he explained, but L's body clearly was prone to do everything on overdrive for no apparent reason, and her symptoms were consistent with MCAS. MCAS caused not only allergic reactions, but the general sense of "feeling off" that L had described. Allergic reactions can come and go with MCAS, with something to which she had never been allergic causing a reaction one day but not the next. L had not had any anaphylactic reactions, but he prescribed EpiPen for us to have on hand should an emergency arise. We kept one on her nightstand, one on my nightstand, one in her backpack, and one with Mia, our beloved Nanny who was a second mom to L and who cared for her as if L were her own. Dr. Gary also prescribed a little-known antihistamine called ketotifen for her to take daily.

June 1, 2017, 11:00 am (age 14)

My phone was always on when I was in meetings with clients. If L, a doctor, or anyone from my house called, I would answer immediately, no questions asked. When my phone rang that morning I grabbed it and quickly excused myself from the meeting I was in.

"She had a seizure while I was sitting next to her on her bed."

I stepped back into my meeting, grabbed my belongings, apologized profusely, and headed straight to the hospital where I would meet L. By the time I arrived at the hospital, all the blood work had come back and did not show any anomalies. The next day would be spent doing various EEGs and other neurological tests, all of which showed nothing that would cause a seizure. The doctors at the hospital didn't have an explanation, but Dr. Gary thought it could be a reaction to the ketotifen. He hadn't seen this type of reaction before, but then again, he hadn't seen anyone quite like L before either, and it was the only thing that had changed in her treatment. One incident was enough in his mind, so we were done with ketotifen. Not worth the risk. Off the ketotifen, it would be almost a year before L would have another seizure.

"What do we do to manage the MCAS?" I asked "Daily Claritin, for now," he said.

"That's it? That seems too simple."

"It probably is, but hopefully we won't need to go the more complicated route. And, yes, there is a more complicated route. Let's start here and see what happens."

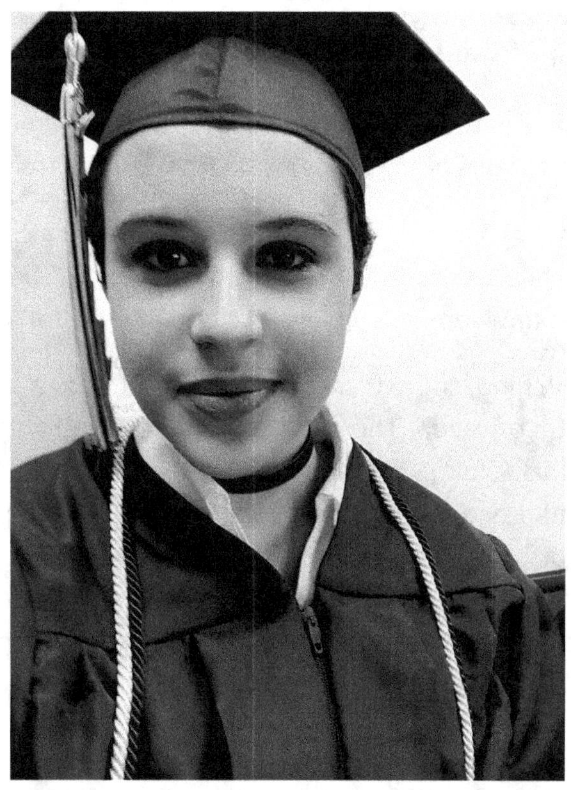

L's 8th grade graduation, June 6, 2017, age 14.

June 25, 2017 (age 14)

"Hey, Mom, can you come look at this?"

L showed me her left foot. Right on top of her foot, an irregular shape about a half-inch long started to faintly take shape. It looked as if the very top layer of skin had been scraped off, and a layer of raw, new, pink skin was peeking through.

"How did this happen? Did you scrape yourself?"

"No, Mom, I've literally just been sitting here."

"Does it hurt? I mean more than your baseline pain?"

L looked at me the way teenagers look at their parents when it is clear that the parents are just clueless, "What do you think?"

Within about 10 minutes, three more of these abrasions appeared on her foot while we were just sitting there talking. They seemed to emerge out of nowhere.

By that evening, there were two more, and by the next morning she had a total of seven. They had become raw and were oozing an orangey, reddish fluid. Dr. Gary tried to stay upbeat when I called him, but I could hear the concern in his voice. "What are we going to do with our girl?" he asked out loud. He let out a big sigh, "Take her to a dermatologist and see what they say. In the meantime, it is imperative that these lesions not get infected. I'm calling in several prescription antibiotic ointments to your pharmacy. Go pick them up. Now."

 The dermatologist had no idea what was causing the lesions. He instructed us to keep them clean and to keep them safe from infection. "Thanks a lot," I thought to myself. "I know that, but can someone please tell us why they are spontaneously emerging and how we prevent them?" We never did get an answer to that question.

Over the next few months, the lesions took on a life of their own. There was a pattern. Before they erupted, L would have a spike in her pain for about two days. Then they would appear, very faint, with just the top layer of skin seeming to erode. Within a few hours they would turn rust-colored and ooze. This stage, L said, was the most painful. After about a week, they would start to scab over, but through the scabs, they would spontaneously start bleeding. A lot. Like, pools of blood. Eventually they would turn into dark purple scars. Sometimes the scars would be dormant, and sometimes they would reopen, starting the whole process again.

The cycle took about a month to complete. And so began another part of L's daily routine. Texting me in the middle of the night to show me new lesions starting, cleaning them, applying antibiotics, wrapping her feet in gauze to prevent her bed from being soaked in blood, and waiting to see when more would show up. By the end of the summer, she had over 40 scars covering both feet, some extending to her calves. The larger ones were three inches long and two inches wide, a permanent reminder of lesions that had healed while new ones continued to creep in.

She wrote and recorded an acapella version of this song the day the lesions began.

Don't Wanna Go
L Grey
June 25, 2017 (age 14)

I don't wanna go
And it hurts to leave
But there's nothing here and I know you'll grieve
But I gotta run
I gotta go
'cross the desert plains Oh don't you know
If I don't leave now
If I don't go
I'll crawl back out
I'll make it home
And I can't die semi-alive
So I gotta run
Say goodbye
I'm not scared
I'm not scared
I'm not scared
I'm not scared
I'm so scared
I'm so scared
But I gotta go

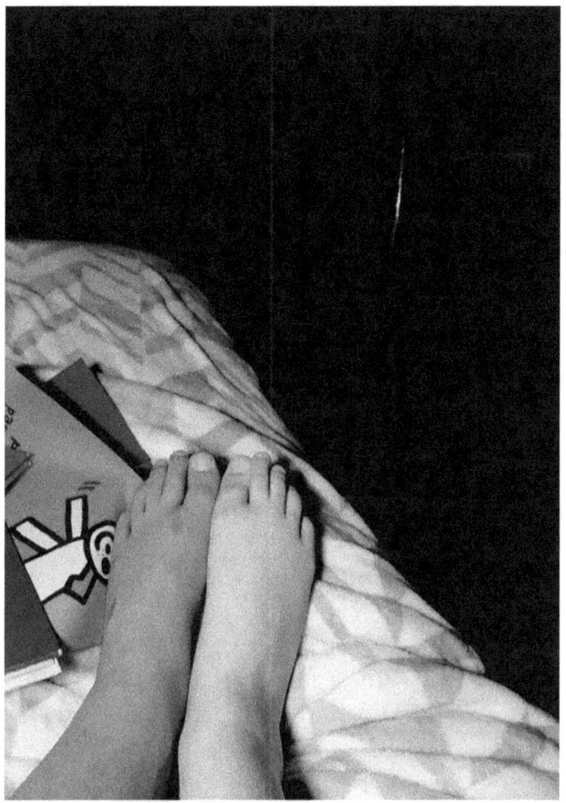

L's first lesions, June 25, 2017, age 14.

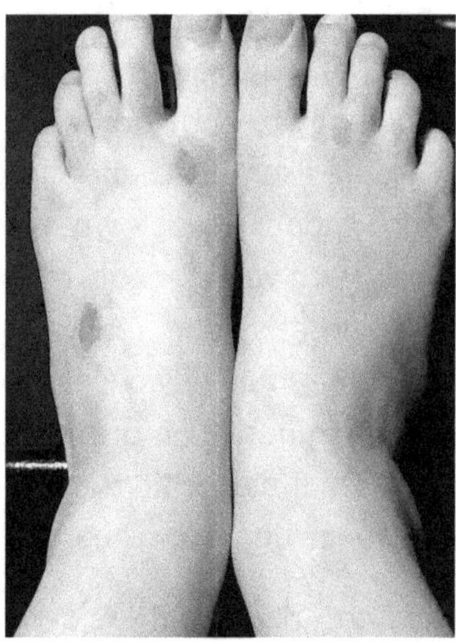

The next morning, June 26, 2017, age 14.

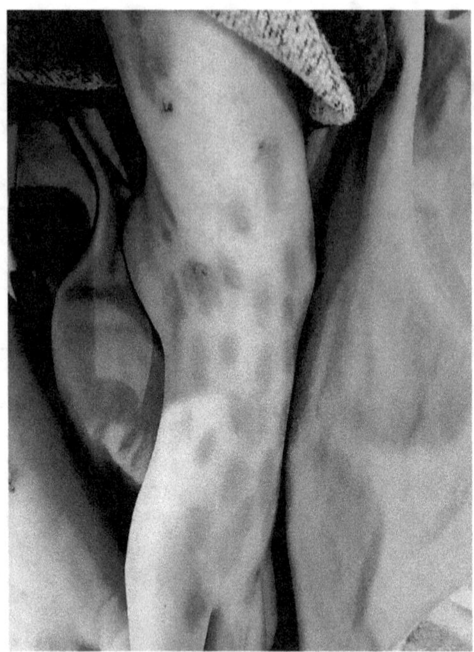

L's scars by May 2018, age 15.

July 2017 (age 14)

The lesions were not going to stop L from going on the trips we planned. With her feet wrapped in gauze and a backpack filled with medication, we made our way to New York, Philadelphia, and Washington, DC. Although we had sent Dr. Gary photos, we both wanted him to see what was going on with his own eyes. He was stumped. He suspected it had to do with vascular constriction caused by CRPS, but he knew that was an unsatisfactory answer for all of us. He also didn't like that L's heart rate remained so elevated, despite her drinking water and Gatorade religiously. He prescribed a beta blocker to see if that would help. When it didn't, he tried another one, and then another. But they didn't touch her racing heart.

From there we went to Arizona, where L was able to maneuver herself onto a raft in a pool and float for a few minutes. Her goal was to swim, but the sensation of water was too unbearable on her skin, and the risk of going in the water with open lesions was too great. That would have to wait. She would feel accomplished with just the float.

Throughout the summer, as her heart continued to race and lesions appeared without warning, she did her best to keep her sister from worrying while she was away at camp. She entertained Jaz with her unique brand of humor, sending Jaz huge close-up photos of some of her favorite historical figures, along with random, little known facts about them. That summer Jaz was flooded with pictures of and stories about Hamilton, Beethoven, Oscar Wilde, and a photo of Ms. K, her math tutor, just because.

L was also planning for the upcoming school year. She would be a freshman in high school. The gifted school that had been so gracious in accommodating her needs only went through eighth grade, so we needed to figure out how to get her through high school. We knew there was no way she could attend school in person full-time, so we enrolled her in a university-backed, accredited online program. Our local high school was incredibly supportive. Because we were in the district, L could take classes at the high school even though she wasn't enrolled full-time. After two-and-a-half years of being homeschooled, L was craving a bit of normalcy and the chance to experience a bit of adolescence. She signed up for an acting class with a renowned teacher whose impact on the community was legendary. The goal would be for her to attend school for 45 minutes a day. As it turned out, she was able to go for one, maybe two days a week through early November. After that, she was unable to return. But the time she spent there filled her with a sense of purpose and belonging.

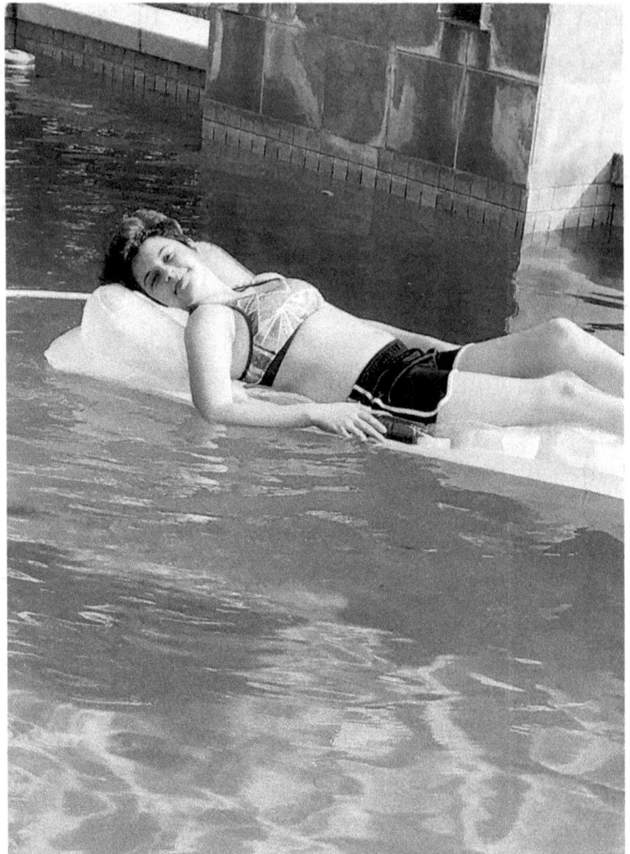

L floating in Arizona, July 24, 2017, age 14.

I've always been a walker. It's been a source of meditation and therapy for me. During the summer of 2017 I walked a lot, as often as I could. My walks were consumed with two things. The first was a knowing that there was an undiagnosed autoimmune component to L's illness. This wasn't a thought or a hypothesis. This was a deep, unequivocal knowing. As L's heart raced, as her feet bled, as her breath became short and her body burned, I knew that her immune system was attacking her. I shared this with Dr. Gary; he did not disagree. The challenge was that neurological autoimmune diseases were notoriously hard to diagnose. There were no commercially available tests, so diagnoses often only came from being part of a clinical trial. And once diagnosed, treatment was uncertain at best. But Dr. Gary and I decided we would leave no stone unturned to try and understand the autoimmune angle. It would be 10 months later, in May of 2018, that we would have our answer.

The second thing that filled my mind during these walks was the image of L's death. I saw it. I saw it all. I saw myself finding her. I saw myself trying to revive her. I saw her funeral. I heard her eulogy in my head. I would squint my eyes and shake my head the way a child does when they do not want to see something, as if in so doing I could make the thought disappear. But it always came back in vivid detail. A year later, the images from my walks played out with chilling accuracy.

August 2017 (age 14)

"When I'm able, there are two concerts I want to go to: Lady Gaga and Stevie Nicks. Gaga because she's wicked smart and a total supporter of the LGBTQ community. And Stevie because she's the coolest person ever. Well, we know she's not really a person. She's a witch. But whatever, that's just semantics. She is tapped in, if you know what I mean."

"Stevie is actually going to be at Ravinia next month," I said. "Why don't we try to go? Ravinia is right here; we can picnic and sit on the grass and leave whenever you want." "Awesome. I'm in."

August 23, 2017 (age 14)

It was the first day of high school. We had been to the school before, and L had scoped out exactly where the elevator was and how she would get to the studio theater where her acting class was. The security guard, Luis, was extraordinarily kind and had given L his cell phone number and told her not to hesitate to call if she ever needed anything. I don't know that I can adequately describe the feelings that washed over me that morning as I watched her wheel into the building with her feet wrapped in gauze, her backpack slung on the back of her wheelchair, and her head held high. I was filled with an overwhelming sense of pride for what she was doing, for what she had endured and would continue to endure, for the courage she showed every day, and for the person she was. And it was coupled with an equally intense feeling of sadness for what I felt should have been, for what I had hoped and dreamed for her. All I could think was "How did we get here? And how on earth is she able to do what she is doing right now?"

"Mom, Shall (the acting teacher's nickname) is amazing. He's one of the few people who actually lives up to the hype. I'm really happy I'm in his class.

And the kids in the class are really cool. No one looks at me funny because I'm in a wheelchair."

"Oh, honey, you made me day," I hugged her. I couldn't help it.

"So, we did this exercise where we had to say, 'I am a girl (or boy) who…' and then we have to fill in the blank with something meaningful about ourselves. It's one of those acting icebreakers like we used to do at Second City. So, I volunteered to go first. I said, 'I'm a girl who came out when she was 10.' I didn't actually think it was that big a deal, but Shall stopped the class and asked everyone to take a moment. 'L just did what I didn't have the courage to do until I was in my mid-twenties. Can we all just think about that for a minute?' Then, everyone in the class, without Shall even asking them to, just stood up and started applauding. So, yeah, it was a good day. It gave me that hashtag-warm-fuzzy-feeling inside."

September 10, 2017 (age 14)

L's lesions were particularly angry that day, but it was the day of the Stevie Nicks concert, and she was determined to hear the live performance. Ravinia music festival is a holdout from a different era. Tucked into our quiet neighborhood in suburban Chicago, it attracts everything from classical orchestras to folk music to old-school rock 'n' roll. The crowds are always peaceful, and you can sit outside and tune out the rest of the world for a few hours.

L carefully wrapped her feet in gauze while I went to Potbelly's to pick up our picnic dinner. A turkey sub for me, and a pizza sub for her with salt and vinegar potato chips and oatmeal chocolate chip cookies for dessert. We made our way to the concert and spread out a blanket, and I lifted L from her wheelchair down to the grass so she could have the full experience. We knew getting back on her chair would be a challenge, and that she'd resist my help, but she and Melissa had been working on how she could hoist herself from the ground back up to her chair, and she had gotten pretty good at it. L knew that an evening out like this would wipe her out probably for three or four days to follow. There would be no physical therapy; she may not even leave her room as her body tried to recover. But it was worth it. We spent the evening looking up at the stars, filling our bellies with some of her favorite foods, and allowing Stevie's enchanting, haunting voice to fill our souls.

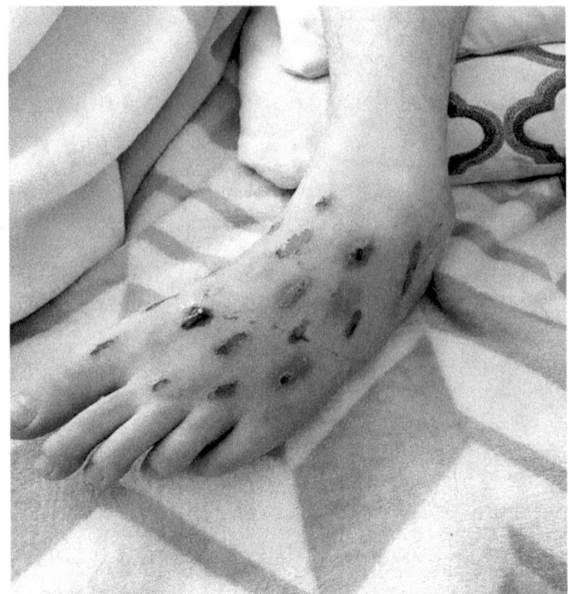

L's lesions the day of the Stevie Nicks concert, September 10, 2017, age 14

September 13, 2017 around 1:00 am (age 14)

The unmistakable ping of the text.

Mom, can you come in?

L was lying on her bed, her left leg shaking uncontrollably, her foot contorted so that it was pointing inward at a 45-degree angle.

"My foot turned in, and I literally can't move it; it's like it has seized in this position. I have no muscle control, and I can't move it out of this position." It was time to see Dr. Lubenow again.

September 17, 2017 (age 14)

L had been wanting to see *Hamilton* for 18 months. She and her friends knew every song lyric, and L being L, she knew the history of Alexander Hamilton and where the musical was true to history and where it took some liberties. My dad got us all tickets with accessible seating as an early birthday present to her. It was a bad pain day; she still hadn't recovered from the Stevie Nicks concert, her foot was still seized, and she had been out of school all week, but she figured she'd have enough adrenaline to make it through the performance —and she did. She ate Swedish Fish and popcorn as she let herself get lost in Lin Manuel Miranda's brilliance. On the surface, the day seemed like a success. A hard-fought success, but a success, nonetheless. That evening, as the stress of the outing wreaked havoc on her body, she penned this poem:

Sunday Melancholy (I cannot exist)

L Grey

September 17, 2017 (age 14)

I cannot exist within this body
This life is not conducive to living
It is suffocating
And overwhelming
And trapping
Not some Sunday Melancholy that can be walked away in a few city blocks
Or a ping of homesickness that goes well with misty streetlights
There is no out running this
There is no leaving

It is suffocating
And overwhelming
And trapping
And lonely
So deeply, untouchably, indescribably lonely.
Lonely in a bone crushing
Soul aching
Archaic torture kind of way;
Not poetic
Or beautiful
Or something to derive strength from
Just lonely.
Just painful.
Survival itself is never far from conscious thought
Staying alive, so that one day
I can look back over the pages I've written
and sigh with relief that the story's been told

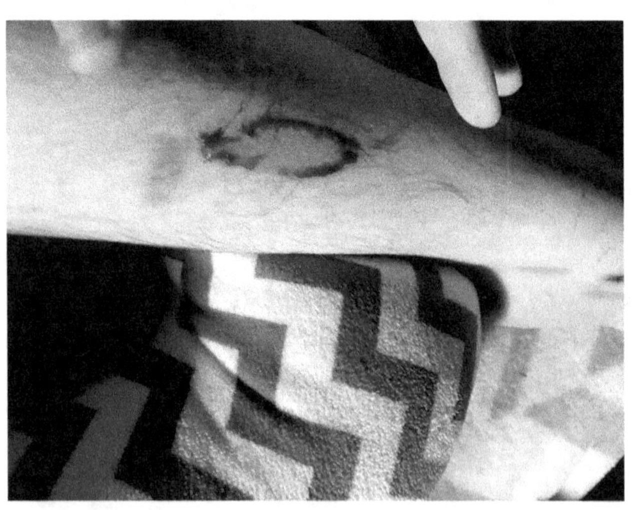

L's lesions the day of Hamilton, September 17, 2017, age 14.

September 18, 2017 (age 14)

We sat in the exam room at Dr. Lubenow's office retelling L's history to the terrified resident who happened to have the misfortune of coming into our room. He was clearly out of his depth. L walked through her history quickly (she had done this too many times) and ended by explaining her lesions and the seizing of her foot.

"Can I take a look?" the resident asked.

"Sure," L said, as she unwrapped the gauze.
"Holy shit," the resident's eyes widened, and he seemed completely unaware that those words had actually come out of his mouth. He left the room quickly. When he regained his composure, he came back, and asked if he could take a picture of L's feet for learning purposes, since he had never seen anything like it before.

"Go ahead," L instructed him. "You'll probably want to see my calves too, there are some big ones there."

We never saw that resident again.

Dr. Lubenow entered the room with his usual calming confidence. He had seen this before, but only rarely, and never in children. He and Dr. Gary had been corresponding, and they both felt that now that L had gone through some extensive detoxing, perhaps we should try ketamine one more time. The rationale was that if the toxins in her body had prevented ketamine from working two years prior, maybe now those channels were clear and the ketamine could break through.

L was ambivalent but ultimately agreed that, at worst, she'd have three days of ketamine misery, a relatively short blip in her now two-and-a-half-year journey.

"Okay," she agreed. "But just that round. If it doesn't work, we're done with ketamine. By the way, tell me honestly, am I like your typical patients? Or am I more extreme?"

He looked solemn and serious. "You've got the most severe, complex, intractable case I've seen."

Her ketamine infusion was scheduled for October 17–19.

October 17–19, 2017 (age 14)

The early morning drive was mostly quiet. I had learned not to try to distract L with meaningless banter when she was preparing for medical procedures. She needed to be in her own head, and the truth was I needed to be in mine. I watched her in the passenger seat, eyes closed, headphones on, wondering what she was thinking. She opened her eyes.

"So, don't freak out when I say this, but if for some reason I don't wake up…"

"L, of course you're going to wake up…"

"I know, I know. But I'm just saying, if for some reason I go all Michael Jackson with the propofol and I don't wake up, you should play 'Another One Bites the Dust' at my funeral. Think about it. It would be epic. You'd play it like a processional at a wedding as people were filing in for the service. And it would be super awkward and uncomfortable because people wouldn't know if it was a joke or if you were serious. Everyone would be looking around thinking that it was super inappropriate but also kinda laughing at the same time, and then they'd be mad at themselves for laughing. It would be so classic. Seriously, Mom, if the anesthesia does me in, you should totally do that."

We got to Dr. Lubenow's office, and L let me hold her hand and pet her head while they prepped her. I gave her a kiss goodnight as the cocktail of ketamine and propofol entered her body, and I sat down for the same vigil I had sat two years prior, this time for three days.

She awoke with the distinct smell of ketamine on her breath, expressing her guilt over being sick and making me promise I wouldn't leave her alone in a forest to fend for herself. She fumbled to find her tongue and navigate it back into her mouth. "Get back in there, bitch," she commanded her tongue.

"Is your pain any better?" I asked.

"Fuck no," she slurred. "This shit never works. That doctor is kinda cute though. A little young for you, but I say go for it, *carpe diem*, ya know!"

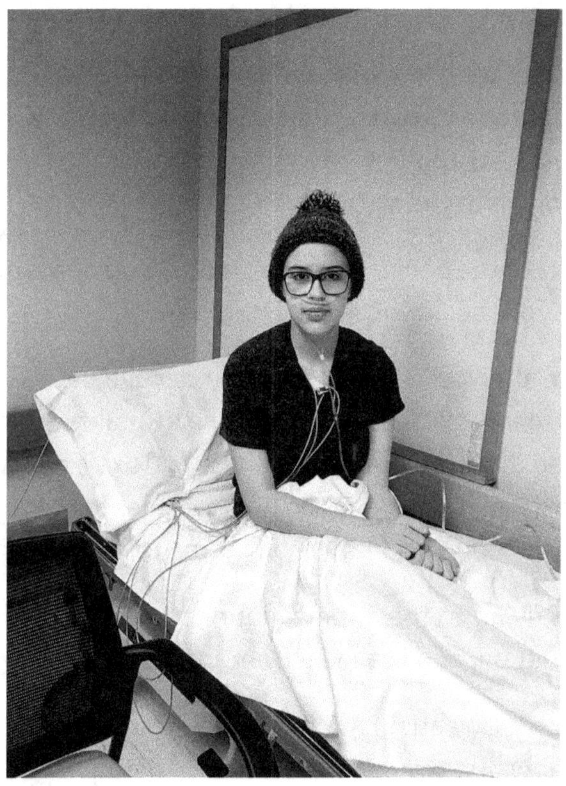

L, prepped for her final ketamine treatment, Oct. 17, 2017, age 14.

November 8, 2017, 1:41 am (four days shy of 15)

I was in Texas on a ranch about 60 miles outside of Dallas running a team session for one of my long-standing clients. L called me in the middle of the night.

"Something is really wrong. I was stretching in my sleep, and I felt and heard the scar on my back where the spinal cord stimulator is rip open. I can't see it, but I can feel that it's open, and it feels like the device is moving in my back. I can feel it."

I texted my dad while she was talking. He would sleep over when I had to travel for work, and he was sleeping down the hall from L. He went in her room while we were talking and was able to take a picture of her back and send it to me. L had described it clearly. The thick scar from the spinal cord implant was torn open, and L had an open wound on her back, down to the muscle.

I tried to keep the panic out of my voice. "Grandpa is going to clean and bandage your back while I call Dr. Lubenow."

I called the after-hours emergency number and packed up my things while I waited for one of Dr. Lubenow's fellows to call me back. When I got the call, I texted the on-call fellow the photo and explained what had happened. "Keep it clean," he said. "Do not bring her to the ER. They won't know what to do. Bring her into the office first thing in the morning."

I started driving to the airport, figuring there would be a 5:00 am flight I could get on, and I called L from the car.

"Don't worry, sweetie. I'm on my way home and we are going to see Dr. Lubenow first thing in the morning. Grandpa is going to stay in your room tonight."

"Mom, I'm okay," she was doing her best to keep me calm. "Grandpa doesn't need to stay in my room. I know he's right down the hall, and I'll call if I need him, but you know I really just want to be alone."

I reluctantly agreed that she could have her privacy. Unbeknownst to her, my dad sat right outside her door for the rest of the night, listening for the slightest sound of distress.

Back in Dr. Lubenow's office, it was clear that the device had dislodged itself and was now sitting in her mid-back, causing her excruciating pain. Why it dislodged, and why a two-year-old scar tore open down to the muscle, we would never know.

"I need to surgically remove the device. We can do it Monday." It was Thursday. There was no way this was waiting four days. I begged him to get her in on Friday. "Please, Dr. Lubenow, please." He rearranged his schedule, and we were set for the next day.

"After she has healed from the removal," Dr. Lubenow explained, "you should consider implanting a new device. It is called a DRG stimulator and it is the most significant development in the treatment of CRPS that I have seen in 15 years. It is new to the market, but I have seen extraordinary results. I think it could be life changing for L."

We tossed around the idea. We didn't like the thought of an additional surgery, or additional hardware in her body, but nothing else had even come close to alleviating her condition. We decided to go for it, and the DRG surgery was scheduled for December 29.

November 9, 2017 (3 days shy of 15)

I emailed Shall to let him know L was having surgery and probably would not be back in school until after Christmas break since her recovery time seemed to be getting longer and longer with each treatment or procedure. I thanked him for his support and for making L's limited high-school experience such a positive one. I still have his response:

I think L is an incredible young woman and have enjoyed every second of our time together. With all the challenges L has faced, she remains bighearted, courageous, and kind. You have obviously provided L the love, support, and tools she needs to know the truth: She is a beautiful human being, worthy, and wise. Please know I am here every step of the way as L's journey continues.

L and I sat in the pre-op area confirming with the various nurses what procedure was going to be done, meeting the anesthesiologists who would be monitoring her, and willing time to go by.

"Mom, I know this sounds morbid, but every time I go in for surgery, I really worry that I won't wake up. I mean, I know these are trained professionals and everything, but I can't help it. And the funny thing is, it's not like my life is so great right now. I'm not exactly living the dream. But I don't want to die because of some surgical fuck-up, like an anesthesiologist who is asleep at the switch, or a surgeon who has shaky hands, or some weird-ass post-op infection. No, man, that's not how I want to go. I have this overinflated ego or something because I really, really want to have an impact on this world. And I'm worried I'm going to die before I can have the kind of impact I know I can have. That probably sounds arrogant, but it's just true. Are you picking up what I'm putting down, Mom?"

"Let's set a couple things straight," I said. "First of all, you are not going to die on the operating table. No way, no how. Not gonna happen. Second, you have already had more of an impact on this world than you could possibly understand. You need to trust me on that."

I squeezed her hand as the nurse came in to give her some Versed, an anti-anxiety drug they give patients before they are wheeled into the OR so they're kind of woozy by the time they arrive.

"Hey, if it's okay, could you not give me any Versed? I've had it a bunch, and I really don't like it. I like to be alert up until the last second."

The nurse looked at me, and I nodded in agreement with L's request. She knew her body, and she knew her mind.

I often thought about this conversation, and many others like it, after her death. It may seem odd that a girl who ultimately made the decision to end her life would be so concerned about her premature death, but with L, it made perfect sense. She was not depressed. She did not want to die by accident before she was ready, before she had determined that she had done all she could possibly do in her body. She wanted to stay in her body for as long as she could. For me, for her sister, for her family, for the words she needed to write, the justice she needed to seek, the causes she need to champion, and the people whose lives she needed to touch. There was so little about her physical condition that she could control, and she'd be damned if, after her long, grueling fight, she would go before her time due to a surgical misstep or a virulent infection.

The removal of the device went smoothly, and L would spend her 15th (and final) birthday, on November 12, in bed recovering from surgery.

"Next year's birthday has to be better," she was half declaring and half pleading.

"It will be," I promised. "It will be."

Christmas Break, December 2017 (age 15)

We were headed to Sanibel for the first time in three years. We had our travel routine down to a science at this point. My dad had rented a house with an elevator, along with one of those wheelchairs with big, inflatable, rubber tires that could go on the sand so that L could make it to the beach and watch the sunset while she listened to the ocean.

We were all together, in the place that felt most like home, trying to ignore the reality of how dire L's condition was. The lesions on her feet were multiplying and bleeding profusely. Her left ankle was still seized at a 45degree angle (it would be permanently stuck this way). The heat made her heart race to almost 200 beats per minute and would cause angry red hives to blossom all over her body, her shoulder was dislocating almost daily, and her pain was unrelenting.

But we were there, and L would put on long sleeves and pants to shield her skin from the sun, and I'd push her rubber-tired wheelchair down the path to the beach, running as fast as I could to make it like a rollercoaster ride, like I used to do when she was a toddler in her stroller. We would watch the sunset and talk about her plans for the future. The surgery to implant the new DRG device was scheduled for the day after we were to return home, and she was nervous about it but also hopeful. She daydreamed about being able to swim the next time we were back in Sanibel and talked about how eager she was to go back to Shall's class when she had recovered from her surgery.

Our time there was emotional. We were grateful to all be together, but we were haunted by happier times. Memories of L and Jaz playing games in the pool, laughing freely, and swimming until their fingers were prunes permeated every moment, and we all longed to go back to that time.

L's time in Sanibel was particularly bittersweet. It was a huge accomplishment for her to be there and something she was determined to do. In retrospect, I am so glad that she was able to make it that one last time. But she was also acutely aware of how different her experience of Sanibel was at age 15, compared to the last time she was there at age 12, before she got sick. She was so close to her happy place yet so very, very far from it.

She would have moments of passion and enthusiasm. She was triumphant when we first wheeled down to the beach and she could see the ocean and hear the waves crash on the sand. She challenged her grandparents to intense games of Bananagrams and Rummikub, and, never one to shy away from a good debate, she would look to challenge her grandpa every chance she got. He was, perhaps, her favorite person to debate. One night, as we were sitting at Timbers for dinner (she had bread and a baked potato), she boldly declared, "Grandpa, you're a racist." My dad looked flummoxed. "But it's okay," she was laughing at this point. "It's not your fault. It's just your generation. You're a 75-year-old white guy. You can't help it. You say things that you don't even know are racist. You're not a bad guy, really, I love you and everything, but you're a racist."

"What kind of things do I say?" he wondered.

"It's just that you continuously discount the institutional racism that exists in this country. There are systems that have been in place for generations that are designed to oppress minorities, and you're clueless about them. But like I said, it's a generational thing. I have a book for you to read, it's called *The New Jim Crow*. Read it, and then we'll talk more."

My dad agreed to read the book, and L shoved a hunk of bread in her mouth. "You're also a misogynist, but we'll cover that tomorrow. I can tell Jaz is getting annoyed by the conversation tonight. By the way, this bread is *real* good. Ten out of ten."

L was undoubtedly glad to have made it there and to have this time with her family, but she was quietly consumed with how much she was suffering, with a legal system that refused to prosecute her abuser, and with increasing dread over her impending surgery.

Entry 1
L Grey
Dec. 17, 2017 (age 15)

I'm not really sure what inspired me to start this journal. It was a spur of the moment thing. Maybe it's because I'm lonely, and a page will always listen. Maybe it's because a page will never talk back or judge, or even understand. Maybe it's my need to be known, to sculpt my own future. Maybe, one day, historians will look back over this diary and say to themselves, "what a tragic life," "what a pity." I don't really know what they'll say. I guess it depends on how things go, and what I write. Maybe I'll publish this, maybe it will never see the light of day. I don't know.

I've written a lot of prose and even more poems. I've written novels, but this is not that. This is unedited. Unscripted. This isn't for the reader, this is for me. This is stream of consciousness.

I don't know why I started this. It certainly wasn't all the shrinks and selfhelp articles telling me to write down my feelings. If I had to guess, I'd say it's a combination of a legacy complex and loneliness.

I'm on vacation right now. Every part of my body hurts. It's screaming. It's dying. If I lay down to sleep I might never get up again. But nonetheless I am going to go down to the beach. The irony is, if I don't, I will be told off for being a shut in. If I do, they will not believe the extent of this pain. But that's hardly a new dilemma. Hell, that's the Chronic Illness Gothic. So I might as well get some sun.

I went to the beach today. We got this big beach wheelchair with giant inflatable tires. There's a certain freedom in looking at the ocean, and a certain restriction of requiring so much assistance to do so. One day, I would like to think that I have a wife or girlfriend, and we go to the beach and have picnics and drink lots of wine. I like to think that she loves me

unconditionally. I am the world's most romantic cynic, I think. I don't expect a storybook love- in fact, I don't think it's even real. But god, It's something to dream about. In my dreams, everything is beautiful and nothing hurts. Then, on other days, I dream I am dead. In the end, the pain-free outcome is the same either way. But alas, that's a dark and off topic thought. I digress.

It's strange and upsetting to think that, the day after I get home, while I am still jet lagged and exhausted, they're going to stick me on a table and cut into my spine. I can feel an ache in my back just thinking about it. The thought of health never really leaves. The thought of survival never really leaves.

I'm going to go now. Maybe sleep a little before dinner. I wrote some prose earlier today. It's not good, but I think I'll leave it here:

"The house is warm. Too warm. There is a certain indescribable stillness that comes with the afternoon heat. As though it is too hot to move or even to think. It is a muggy, mosquito filled quiet. The sun lingering up in the sky, unflinching and unforgiving. It is a heat that brings with it exhaustion and nostalgia.

The house is old. I can feel it's history. There is no rumble of air conditioning to bring a respite from the heat. There is only this forced tranquility that makes limbs feel like lead. Everything moves slower than perhaps it should. In the quiet, in the stillness I longed for, there is pain.

This house is not like the house at home- this house is happy and full.

Suitcases lay scattered all over, with clothes and bathing suits falling out. Towels on the floor and half drunk beers on the counter. There is evidence of joy here. There is evidence of family.

The joy is down by the pool, it is at the beach. From this unbearably stuffy room, I can hear the joy splashing and laughing. I can hear the joy bantering and drinking. Lemonade and swimming pools give the joy coolness. They are not trapped in the silence of afternoon heat. They are not trapped at all. It is just me, having strange, inexplicable heat-induced thoughts.

I have not been on a vacation in years. Sun like this is not conducive to rosetinted memories, it is a light shined on all the things I never wanted to feel again. The family I used to have, the energy. It is almost impossible to remember a time when I did not have to spend whole days in bed. Whole weeks. The bed I am writing this from is probably older than me. The plaque on the wall says this house was built over 170 years ago. I cannot help but wonder if there are any ghosts who are angry their space is now used for vacation rentals. I cannot help but wonder if this tiny, secluded room I am in was once servants quarters. In the cold, I can look back with a sad smile and knowing appreciation. But in the afternoon heat of a foreign place, the past festers."

Entry 2
L Grey
December 23, 2017 (age 15)

They told me not to talk about it. They said I should delete all social media, not mention it to friends. That I had to work hard to maintain my image as the perfect victim. That if I was angry or tired or sad, or too thin or too fat, too sick or too healthy, they would say I am crazy. Say I am nothing but an autistic loon from a broken home.

I want scream "ME TOO". I want to join the movement. I want to stand on the roof and say "He raped me! He fucking raped me and I hope he dies!" But the fancy lawyer in the fancy suits says I can't. Says that until the trial is over, my story is not mine to tell. This story, this body, has been at the mercy of powerful men its whole life. It belonged to my father, it belonged to Him, it belonged to the doctors, and now it belongs to the lawyers and judges. I have spent my whole life on my knees, begging men in positions of authority to believe me. Begging them to get their hands off me. Begging them to stop.

It should not be my responsibility to be perfect. He raped me. He locked me in his cellar, he pinned me against the wall. He licked my skin, stuck his hands inside of me. He made me bleed years before my first period. He slithered his filthy hands under the training bra I wore. I could feel the coldness of his wedding ring against parts of my body I did not even know existed. He did those things. I am not the monster. I am not the one on trial here. But he is out there, living his life as though nothing *has happened. He thinks he is untouchable, while I agonize over every word I say. He is probably out there, eating other girls like the wolf He is. And I call Him "He" with a capital H because I do not say his name. I will not say his name. He is not real. He is not human. He killed something in me that I will never get back.*

I am not the perfect victim. I am tired. I am angry. I do not forgive him. I will never forgive him. I am 15. I am still scared. I am still scared when I hear a bump in the night. I am scared when a doctor touches me. I am scared when anybody touches me. I am scared when I put in a Tampon. I am scared. I am not perfect. Sometimes I want to kill myself, and sometimes I want to kill him. I am flawed, and I am angry, and I scared, but that does not make me a liar. He raped me, and it should not be my job to clean up the mess he left in his wake.

He raped me. He raped me. He raped me. I was 10 years old. I was a child. He lured me down and he fucked me. It hurt. It hurt so fucking bad. It hurt like nothing ever had before. I have never written about it before- at least not this vividly. In all the shrinks and all the cops, I have never written about it before. I have never talked about the pain. In all the surgeries and all the illness, nothing has ever come close to hurting like his fingers hurt. Five years and I can still feel him inside me. I can still smell his breath. I can feel his tongue against my skin. I didn't tell the cops the full extent of what he did to me. I have not told anybody. It's too late to tell them now. It's too late, but I will always know. I will forever feel it.

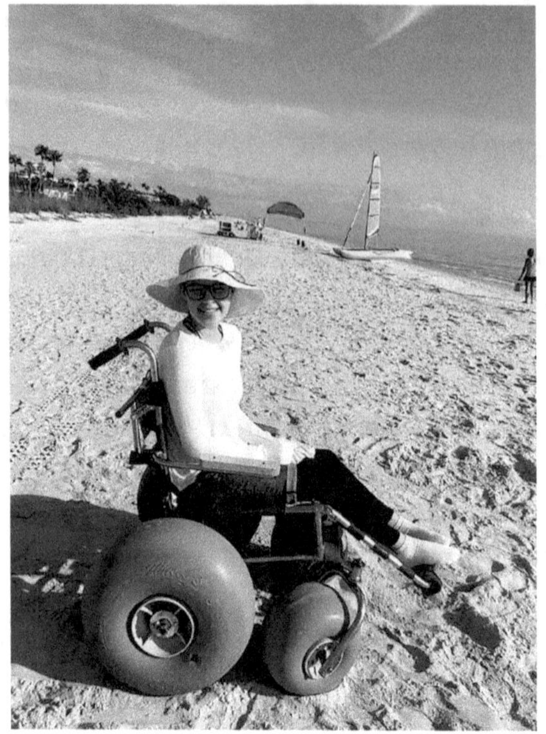

L at the beach in Sanibel, December 2017, age 15.

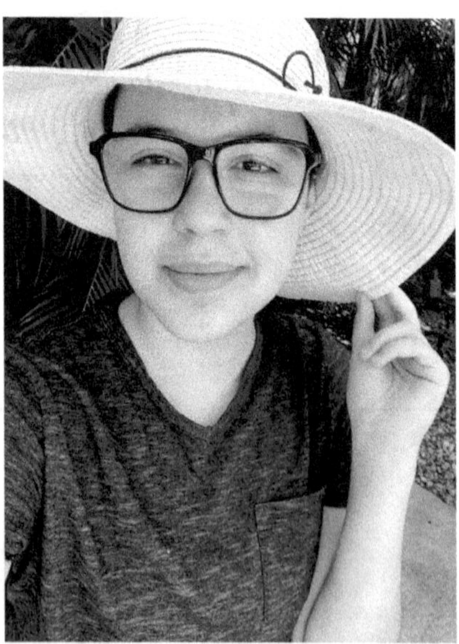

L, self-portrait in Sanibel, December 2017, age 15.

L and I flew home on December 28th. Her surgery was scheduled for the 29th.

Jaz was going to stay in Sanibel through New Year. She might as well stay in Florida with her grandparents; there was no point in her coming home since L and I would be in the hospital. We hugged everyone goodbye and flew to Chicago, hopeful and nervous for what the next day would bring.

December 29, 2017 (age 15)

It was bitter, bone-chillingly cold as we left the house in the darkness of the predawn hours to get to the hospital. L took my hand in the car, "I love you, momma."

"I love you too, baby girl."

That's all we said.

We began our familiar pre-op routine; the nurses, who all knew us at this point, were struck by L's poise, maturity, and stoicism. I snapped a picture just before they wheeled her into the OR, her hair in a shower cap, a smile forced on her lips, and her fingers flashing the peace sign.

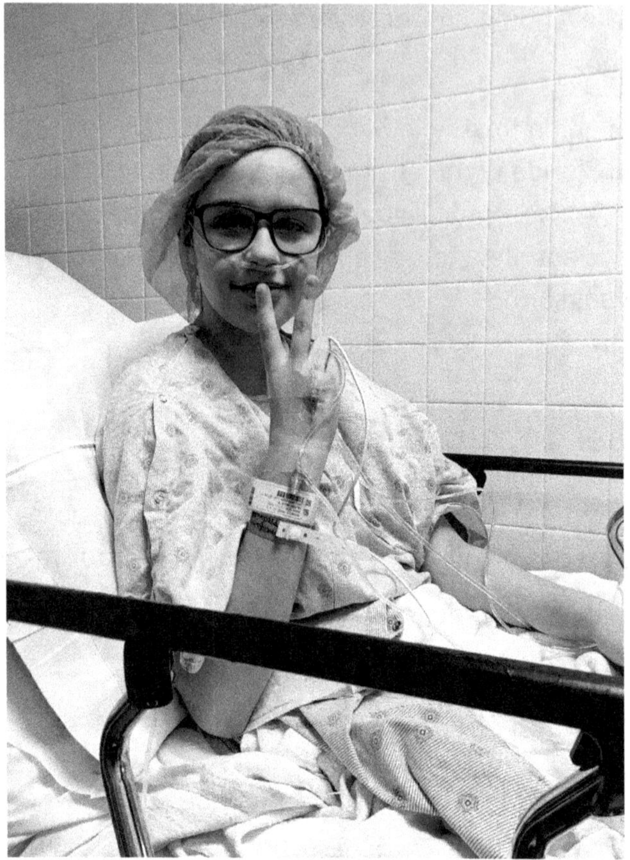

L heading into surgery, December 29, 2017.

I took my seat in the waiting room, knowing it would be at least two-and-a-half hours before I would hear any news from the doctors. I read *People* and *Us* magazines to distract myself and fielded texts from well-meaning family members who were asking for updates long before I would have any. Two-and-a-half hours turned into three, which turned into three and a half, and I willed my mind to quiet itself. Finally, Dr. Lubenow appeared.

"How is she?" I asked.

"The surgery went fine. She's in recovery, but the nurses aren't quite ready for you to go back there. They'll call you back soon."

I didn't like not being in recovery with her when she came to, but there was not much I could do. About 30 minutes later, the nurses called me back to recovery.

"Hi, baby girl," I whispered, trying to mask my anxiety.

L turned her groggy eyes to look at me. I had seen many looks in L's eyes before, but none quite like this. The look she gave me was one of pure, unadulterated terror.

"What is it sweetheart?" I asked. Before she could respond the nurse was giving her a bolus of fentanyl and her eyes rolled back in her head.

"What is going on?" I demanded more than asked.

"She's complaining of pain in her back and her right arm, but I'm sure it is just from the surgery. The fentanyl will help. She should be okay when she wakes up."

As the fentanyl wore off and L came to, the panicked look returned to her eyes, and she looked at me pleadingly.

"Something is wrong, Mom," her words were slurred but her thoughts were perfectly clear. "I've had surgery before, and I know what surgical pain is. This is not surgical pain. This is nerve pain. This is CRPS pain. It's radiating from my right shoulder through my right hand, and it is radiating through my lower back."

L and I both knew exactly what this meant. Not once throughout the course of L's illness had her pain retreated once it spread. We were now looking at the CRPS not only being in her legs, but in her back and her right arm as well. It was an almost unimaginable thought to hold in our heads, and we did not say anything. We just looked at each other while I held her left hand.

"Will you pet my head?" she innocently asked. I perched myself by her bed and pet her fuzzy, buzz-cut head while planting kisses on her forehead as she drifted in and out of consciousness.

Dr. Lubenow came by and tried to offer reassurance that the pain in her arm was likely due to the position of her arm during surgery, and that the pain in her back was surgical. Still, just to be safe, he suggested putting her on a 72hour low-dose ketamine drip to prevent CRPS spread. This would require a transfer to the Pediatric ICU (PICU), as ketamine drips needed to be monitored round the clock. Even though this dose would be nowhere near the massive infusion she had had previously and she would be fully conscious, it needed to be monitored just the same.

L needed to pee, so as the nurses prepared the bedpan, I stepped to the other side of the curtain. It was the first moment I had out of her line of sight; I put my hands over my face, and I cried, uncontrollably. Dr. Lubenow, who was typically rushing from one patient to the next, saw me and came over to try to soothe me. He took my hand and squeezed it with the firm grasp of someone who is used to conveying confidence, even in the most difficult of circumstances. He held my hand for a long time.

As they were preparing to transfer us to the PICU, I called my friend, the physician at the Mayo Clinic in Arizona whom we had visited in the spring. He was an eternal optimist and had always been a sounding board and source of strength for me. I did not expect him to answer. It was the middle of the day, and he carried a full patient load. It was rare for him to answer any calls until late in the evening, but on December 29th he answered on the first ring.

"What's up, V?" his voice calm and soothing from 1,800 miles away. I opened my mouth but found I couldn't form words. Only muffled sobs escaped from my lips. He was patient with me, as he always was, and he waited in silence on the phone until I could choke out words.

"I'm terrified," I kept crying over and over.

"I know you are." There was a quiet gentleness in his words that helped my breathing settle into something that resembled a rhythm.

"She's going to be okay. She's going to be just fine." I don't know if he actually believed that, but his voice was so tranquil, and whether he believed it or not, he knew it was what I needed to hear, if only to get me through the next 24 hours.

It was dark by the time we were settled into the PICU, the machines beeping incessantly and a steady stream of nurses coming in to check L's vitals.

I called Dr. Gary to tell him what was happening.

"Shit," was his response. He had taken a paternalistic role in L's life, and he let out a deep sigh of concern.

"You know my fear," I implored him to tell me something I hadn't thought of.

"I know... I know." Like us, he was a relatively nonobservant Jew. "I think maybe it's time we both found religion. Praying can't hurt."

We would spend the next three days in the PICU, with friends and family trickling in to bring food and flowers. We would duck out of L's room when the nurses helped her to the bathroom, and I would quietly cry in their arms. I felt a desperation present that had not been there before, and I couldn't shed it. Nor could I really describe it. Even as I write this, I struggle to find the words to describe it, just as I struggled then. I would spend the next seven months talking to very few people. It wasn't because I was trying to shut people out, it was just that I lit-erally had no words to describe what was happening to L and to me, both physically and emotionally. This text exchange with a good friend captures it well:

Him: *Happy to be an ear; you can vent or whatever you need.*

Me: *Thank you, I'd vent if I had the words, I just can't seem to find them.*

Him: *Yeah, there are no words for primal feelings.*

New Year's Eve came, and 2017 slid into 2018 with heart-rate monitors blinking, nurses scurrying, and ketamine slowly and steadily dripping into L's veins. At midnight I kissed her cracked, chapped lips and cradled her cheek in my hand. "Happy New Year, baby girl."

"Happy New Year, Mom. I love you."

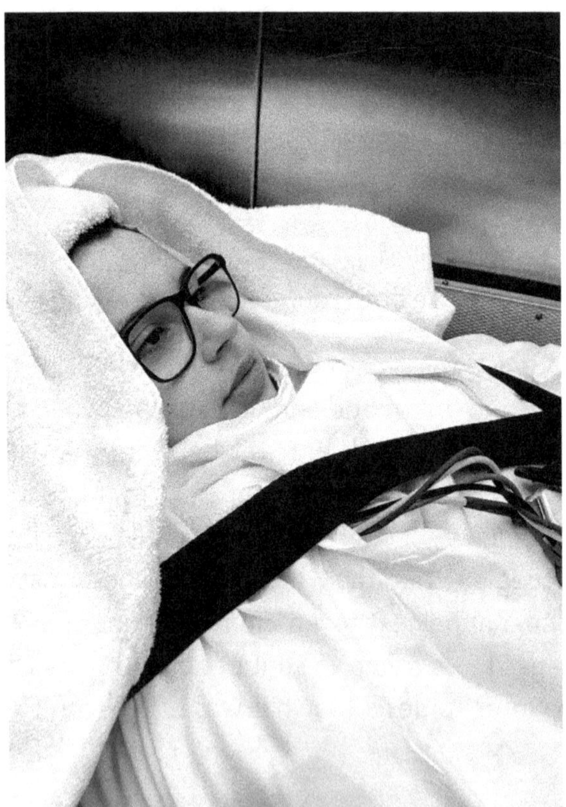

L being transferred to the PICU, December 29, 2017.

January 1, 2018 (age 15)

Entry 3
L Grey
January 1st, 2018 (age 15)

The more time I spend in hospitals, the less human I become. The loudness of the ICU drowns out my voice. Every drop of blood on a scalpel holds a little piece of me that I will never get back. I refuse to let IV's become me. I am at war with PICC lines trying to steal my personality. I never really knew how much of me was based on flannels and cute jeans until I was confined to a hospital gown. In a morphine haze, I told the nurse I would rather starve than let them place a feeding tube. They did not listen, and now there is some foreign entity in my nose running calories into me. There is so much fear I want to spin into poems but I cannot string together a single coherent thought thanks to all the Fentanyl they've given me. The ICU nurse told me last night that the ER sees lots of drunken injuries on New Year's Eve. I wish I was wearing my own clothes, waiting in a crowded ER with my friends, waiting to get stitched up before going back out into the city to live it up. I wish I was there because of a wild night, not because of a mutinous body. I'm scared that by the time they measure every inch of my body for a new custom powerchair, it won't be my body they are measuring. It will be too thin and too otherworldly. The name on the pill bottles, the name my crying mom calls me, is not my name. I am scared that this wrong name, written all over insurance cards and prescriptions, will eat me up. I am scared that I will die more of a curiosity to eager med students than a human being.

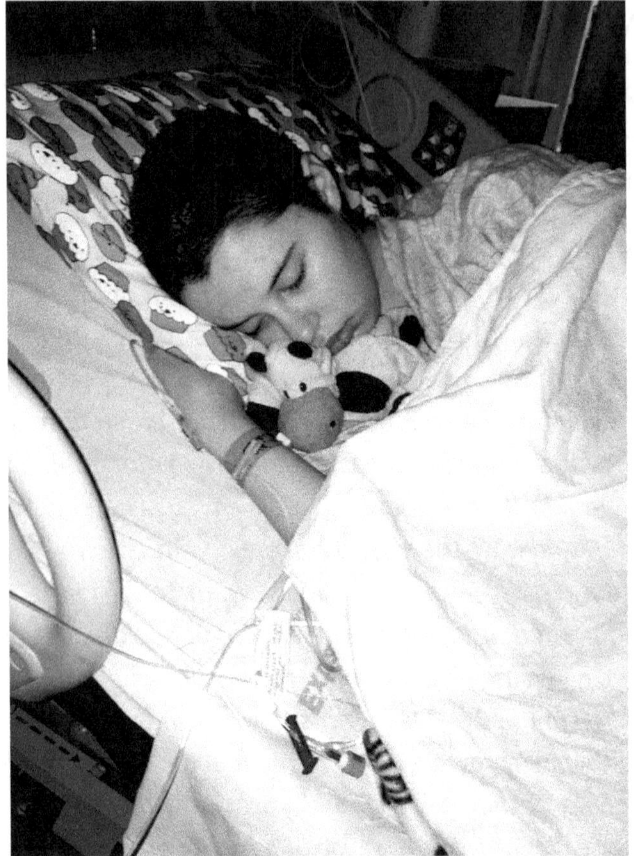

L, New Year's Day, 2018.

January 2, 2018 (age 15)

The pain in L's shoulder and upper arm seemed to be subsiding a bit and, although her right hand was still on fire, the doctors took it as a good sign that her upper arm was doing better. They decided to release us since there was nothing more the hospital could do for us. Time, they said, would be the best healer.

We drove home in the same frigid Chicago winter air that stung us when we arrived, but the cold had become so much more bitter than it had been just three days before.

When we arrived home we got L settled in her bed, trying to make her as comfortable as possible, the unknown future casting a dark shadow over us. Aside from the occasional mandatory trip to the doctor, she would not leave that bed again during her lifetime.

January 3-February 2018 (age 15)

Time had become a blur. L's back pain was so severe that she could not sit up. She would spend the few hours of daylight each day that winter drifting in and out of fitful sleep, her body too exhausted to do much. We would bring food up to her on the days when she had an appetite, and Jaz and I would eat dinner in her room and stay until it was clear she couldn't tolerate company any longer. Her doctors told us to be patient, and we were trying, but we were not seeing any improvement, and the threat of what her future would entail was looming large.

Entry 4
L Grey
January 7th, 2018 (age 15)

I know I should write about the important stuff - the fact that I had surgery, the fact that the surgery went wrong, how I spent my New Years in the ICU. How I've been bedridden since getting home. How my right hand is affected. I will, I'll write about it all. But it's too recent, too real. Even just writing factually about it is too much right now. I want to write it all down, because I know between all the drugs and all the pain, I'll forget these weeks, they'll be lost to the erasure via drugs and trauma. But I am too tired to write about the important stuff. I am too tired to write about anything these days.

The days were dark, literally and figuratively, and I was desperate for anything that might bring some light into her world. She and her best friend, Wes, had often talked about trying to visit each other (he lived outside of Pittsburgh), but when you are sick and disabled, that becomes exceedingly difficult. Like many of her friends, she and Wes met online and had never actually shared the same physical space. This did not diminish their friendship in any way. Their connection was deep and real. I called Wes and asked if he would allow me to fly him to Chicago to visit and to be an extra set of hands to take care of L. The look on L's face when we opened the door to her room and she saw Wes for the first time is one that makes me smile to this day. It was exquisite. They hugged and cried for a long time; the gift of being able to hold each other in the flesh was not lost on either of them. Wes stayed for over a week and came back again in the spring. He brought her food. They listened to music. They did each other's make-up. They took goofy pictures. His gentle, loving, and compassionate energy buoyed L through her darkest days. Wes is part of the family now, whether he likes it or not!

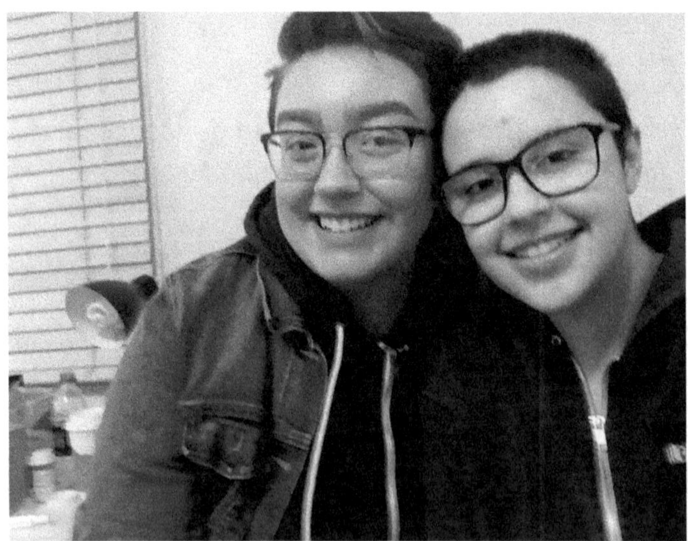

Wes and L, January 11, 2018, age 15.

January 13, 2018, 1:07 am (age 15)

The familiar ping of a text coming through.

Can you come in?

"Can you look at the incisions on my back? They feel weird."

She rolled to her side and I shined my flashlight so I could see the incisions on her back. Her shirt was soaked with blood and stuck to her back. As I peeled her shirt back, I saw five raw incisions that had completely opened down to the muscle and were oozing blood and a sickening orangey-type of fluid. Wes came in and kept her company while I went to CVS to get dressings for the wounds, waiting for the on-call physician to get back to me with further instructions. I sent photos to the responding doctor, who instructed me not to take her to the ER. He told me how to dress the open incisions and insisted on seeing her first thing in the morning.

Getting her to the hospital was a challenge. It was torture for her to sit, even for a minute, and the vibrations of the car sent electric currents through her body. To my surprise, the doctors did not re-stitch her incisions. One of the symptoms of L's EDS was slow healing and the inability of her skin to repair itself. Re-stitching, I learned, posed a greater threat than letting the wounds heal on their own. This, I learned, is why the doctor on call did not want us to go the ER and risk being treated by a doctor who might not understand the implications of EDS on wound healing. They sent us home with clear instructions on how to keep the area clean to prevent infection. That was all they could do. L returned to her bed, and we added the thrice-daily practice of cleaning her incisions to her medical routine. They remained open and slippery for weeks.

L's spirit, while buried under so many layers of pain, worry, and uncertainty, could not be crushed. Her moments of energy didn't last long, but she extracted every ounce from them that she could. Unable to write as much as she previously had (she would type as a form of physical therapy, but between the pain and the fatigue, she was not as prolific as she normally was), she decided to start a podcast. She was determined to have a voice and to use it to try to bring about change. She ordered a microphone and began a podcast series designed to offer support to the disabled community. She titled it *Not Your Inspiration*. It quickly became recognized by iTunes as a new and noteworthy up-and-coming podcast.

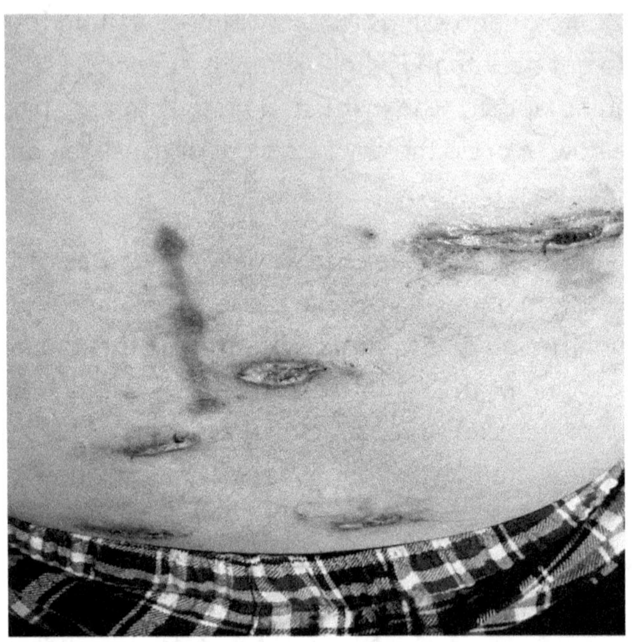

L's open incisions, January 13, 2018, age 15.

Entry 5
L Grey
January 20th, 2018 (age 15)

A lot has happened, and I am, of course, awful at keeping up with this journal. Wes came for a week, which was amazing. Having company and a friend was such a blessing, honestly. He just left 3 days ago, but it feels like longer. My sense of time is so skewed- 5 minutes feels like 20, a day feels like a few hours, a few hours feels like a day, everything is so off. But I digress. It was amazing to meet my best friend for the first time. He was a shining glimmer of light in a sea of shit and sickness.

I'm still stuck in bed. I'm going crazy. I haven't even been able to write- no poems, no journaling, no nothing. I've been fuzzy from the meds and sleeping 18 hour days. I'm exhausted and I can't think. I've never been this tired before. There's never been this much pain before. I think the world thinks I'm lazy and don't want to get up. Fuck that. I hate this. I want out of these four walls more than anybody else. I'm the one stuck in this room, and stuck in this body. I want out more than anybody who says I'm not trying hard enough. Fuck them. The pain is indescribable. It's so hot it's glowing white and red and it breaks through every pill I take. And I take a lot of pills perhaps more than I should. It doesn't matter. My mind is numb and blank. My body is not. I still cannot even sit up. I want out

About a week ago, when Wes was still here, the stitches in my back gave way, and all of the surgical wounds ripped open down to the muscle. Contrary to popular belief, the worst part about this was not the pain or the emergency hospital trip, it wasn't even asking my best friend whom I had just met for the first time in person to carry me into the hospital. No, the worst part is not being allowed to shower. Showering makes me feel human, and without it, I don't know what to do. My skin is greasy beyond belief. My hair is matted down in strange ways. I feel filthy. I am filthy.

I've decided to start a podcast about disability. If you can even call it a podcast- I don't know how to edit audio, and I'm not going to pay to host it on the Podcast app, so it will just be me rambling into a cheap mic on youtube. I'm excited about it though. My biggest fear is dying forgotten, totally unknown, so, if nothing else, I'll leave behind a podcast. I want to write more, I have so many more thoughts buzzing around my brain and begging to come out. I have so much to say, but my thumb is about to dislocate and I'm too tired. I'll be back, sometime.

As January turned to February, the toll that L's illness was taking on every part of her being was clear.

Entry 6
L Grey
February 3rd, 2018 (age 15)

I am going crazy. It's been over a month now, in this room. In this bed. So much of it is blur. I knew this would happen- I knew the drugs and the trauma would corrupt my memory of this past month beyond recognition, which is part of the reason I've been so keen on journaling it. But I haven't written nearly as much as I originally intended too.

I am lonely. There are star stickers on the ceiling above my bed. They've been there since I was 4 years old, and nobody has been able to get them down. They used to glow in the dark, but they haven't in years. Having nothing but star shaped stickers on the ceiling as company is hardly ideal. Of course, I've been in contact with friends. Wes and Agatha and Pashi (I'm sort of dating Pashi now, it's a bit complex, but I digress.) It's pain to talk to them, watch their lives move on without me, watch the world keep turning. I am nothing more than a witness to life. This isn't living, this is surviving.

People have been coming to see me. Christina, my mother's friend, stayed this weekend. Grandparents, friends, the works. I feel like an old Victorian invalid, with guests coming into a dusty sickroom to dispose pity and advice and sympathy. Then sometimes a doctor comes and lays out all their equipment, talking over me to mistress of house, standing over the sickbed and taking note. Seriously, that's what it is. Like I'm some pitiful character in a Jane Austen novel who's taken to bed with TB. So many people, in and out, in and out, all the time. Mom, Jaz, physical therapists, doctors, Sharon (my lovely shrink). It does not stop. They all come in, say somethings, do somethings, and most of the time I stare blankly, almost unaware of what I say in response- totally and utterly dissociated. Then they leave, and I am alone again. There is finally quiet, but it is a lonely quiet.

And sure, I have the podcast, and I have friends who message and call me every day, but I want to go out. I want to go outside. I want to see a movie and go to dinner, take Pashi on a date, live a little. I miss Shall's class and the gang at school. It's going to be spring soon, and I want to feel spring on my face. Hopefully when the power chair comes, I can get out. But that's uncertain, and at best another two months wait.

Ok, my hands are aching and my eyes are closing. Goodbye for now

---

As I read through all of L's writings, it was clear that there were certain days when her existential crisis was more acute than others. May 29, 2016, had been one of those days, and as it turned out, so had February 3, 2018. In addition to the journal entry above, she would open and re-read every poem she had written since her illness began, as if creating a mental log of the progression of her disease, tracking how things could have possibly gotten as dire as they had. And somehow, on that day and in those that would immediately follow, she found the strength to create even more.

Cannot Be
L Grey
February 3, 2018 (age 15)

I don't know
Can't tell you who these shaking hands belong to
I never wanted to know
I didn't plan on the pain
Oceans and oceans of eyes
Every tidal wave of adrenaline
Surfing down cracks in the pavement
Begging for a quick and sterile mercy
I never wanted to see
They say to never whisper the words "this cannot be" after dark
How is this my life?
It condemned me
The agony of an outsider's view
I am no tragic hero
This simply cannot be
They say to remind yourself that this is real
This is real
But there is smog in every corner of my gaze
This is real
I can't see past the rising smoke
This is real
I cannot breathe
This is real
It cannot be
I did not ask to be angry
I am
I will be Who is this
identity?

They say to never ask who you are
But dear lord
Who is this body?
Somewhere in the pride
Somewhere amongst the tumble weeds
This is why they tell you not to look
Close your eyes and count to three
Deep breath in, deep breath out
Little poke-
They told me "don't ask why"
This simply cannot be

Fever Dreams
L Grey
February 3, 2018 (age 15)

Fever dreams make walls dance
But they make this body weak
Fever dreams I can't escape How
long can you stand the heat?
Fever dreams of fear and pain
Hymns of another life
I know just what it's like to die
Embers shaded gray
Avid lovers gone insane
Fever dreams rise and rise
Smoke from other flames
Fever dreams of massacre
Bathwater running red
Fever dreams I won't ignore
And sleep, at last, again

Veins

L Grey

February 7, 2018 (age 15)

Been a long road
Tumultuous way
This house aches greater than the walls could explain
If you squint hard enough there are stars on the ceiling
Scrape them away and it's dark again
Something to be said for old wood flooring
I am every creak
I am every pang
We're growing older
I'm sleeping months away
The weaker we get
Faster life runs
What a travesty I'll die with survival in my veins
I was bred to live with stories on my tongue
When we're gone they'll paint 'em over grey
Burning down old prisons
Doesn't mean there were no captives
Cremate remains
Just to say there was no living
All the bleeding that I've done
Just to be forgotten
Such lament in these floor boards
But they are cool against my face
Never say I did not sing
Never say I did not scream
Just too many words in fragile little veins

How to Write Morphine a Love Song
L Grey
February 8, 2018 (age 15)

Lose yourself to the illness
Crumble
You are an ancient church
Your body is dirty stone
Your body is broken imagery
Archeologists'll dig you up after it is too late
Let yourself surrender
White flag's raised
Sleep now darling, you can mourn tomorrow
Relinquish to the pain
It is all you are
A febrile dream
A scream in the night
Allow the agony to consume you
This sickness is malignant
Your soul will beg for company through the night
Your mind will beg for death
You must deny it
Stay alive
Stay lucid
Next you must wail
Spend your time keeping nurses busy
You are stronger than those dreams
Lie to yourself
You don't need it
Sob the sterility away until you are out of breath
Let your jaw ache from gritted teeth
White knuckles don't make you a saint
Denial's your addiction
You don't need it, you're not sick enough

Pick at the IV
Say a prayer
Sometime before morning it's time to give in
You'll be out before the sun is up
One push and you are an ocean
Tranquil and far out
Deep and dark and unknown Simple blue nothingness
But you'll still feel the panic
You'll still feel the pain
Sickness is a malignancy
It will slither through the thin drug haze
Angels don't wear scrubs
Angels do not slice you open It's just an illusion
Everything is an illusion now
You will lose your pen, your paper, your writing hand
Kiss metaphors goodbye
You are delirious, my dear
You're going to die
This is when you say enough
Rip the needle out
Sleep til you find sanity It will come back
It will always come back
Hold a pill between your teeth
Tell it you're kissing it
You're praying again
Beg the pill to work
Coerce it
This is where you tell the drugs how much you love them
You hate them
They do not work
Lie to them
Tell them they matter

Tell them they are all you have left
All that you are
You're not addicted, honey, you're just sick
Intravenous salvation
You're nothing more than hollowed cheeks and weary eyes
You feel nothing
You think everything
Every breath, every buried scream
This pain itself is Morphine's love song

10,000
L Grey
February 8, 2018 (age 15)

Ten thousand dirt roads
A craving to roam
Yet here we are
Together alone
These are the years that should be missed
We'll look back and say
How did we live
Nostalgia ain't for us
No memories rose tinted
When you recover
Forget me and run
I'll remind you of now
Live on and forgive
Ten thousand acres
Of unexplored woods
I need some time
I need to think
I want to scream but I can't get away
Go into the trees and berate God for this
I'm tied to the bedpost

Bound with silence
When you learn how to sing
In the dead of night
You'll have to go
Tackle down dawn
Ten thousand minutes
And all of them crawling
I want to be reckless
Now's the chance to be careless
We can't go
I know
You're the master caring
We're the saviors
We're damned
Hearts breaking for adventure we'll never have
Let's plan our demise
I'll love you for always
But I won't call you back Plot your escape
That house won't own you
Go fast or face fear
I'll rot
And I'll rot
We can bloom in the snow

Oasis

L Grey
February 18, 2018 (age 15)

Giving up is a mirage
There is no oasis on the horizon It's not real water I see
But oh, how it gleams in the sun
Never before have I been so thirsty
So close is a pond of cool salvation

My lips are chapped and flaking
I am ravenous for change
Parched
I know better than to try and chase down
The mythical place where earth meets sky
That thin line where water lays
Don't run down fever dreams
Never follow delusions of the afternoon heat
I will not die alone
Halfway to hell on a dusty desert road
My obituary will not read
Died in vain
Trying to catch an illusion
Yet in these scorching days
It is a comfort to know
There is a pool on the horizon

One of the many remarkable things about L was that she could momentarily pull herself out from the clutches of fire and temporarily suspend her deep knowing that this disease would not ever release its grip on her. Whether this suspension was for her benefit or mine, I am not sure. It was probably for both. But in between journal entries and poems that expressed her innermost pain, she would allow herself to fantasize about her future. Some of these daydreams had a semblance of reality—she would talk about going to college, living on a farm with her wife, writing poetry, and fighting for social causes. Some of the daydreams were purely fantasy, providing a minute's respite from the daily task of survival.

The Winter Olympics took place in February, and L, in her quest to do everything possible in the world, wondered aloud how she might be able to become an Olympic athlete. Now mind you, she was not completely out of touch with reality, and she knew that sports that required a high degree of athleticism probably wouldn't work really well for her. She started to brainstorm the most obscure Paralympic events she could participate in. She figured curling did not take a great degree of physical strength and she could wheel around on the ice, sweeping it vigorously with her broom. Still, given that she had no experience, she reckoned it might be hard to earn a spot on the US team. She'd need to join a team that was not known for its winter sports. That's when it hit her. As a Jew, she could automatically join the Israeli team, and, she figured, there couldn't possibly be that many wheelchair-bound Israeli curlers—surely she could make the cut! Problem solved; she had a plan! We laughed mightily at the image of her moving to Israel to train with the Paralympic curling team, and I promised her I'd be at the rink cheering her on like a maniac. In the coming months, we'd come back to that image, as a reminder to both of us that we could still laugh. And laugh we would. She had also discovered a Hungarian rendition of "Who am I" from *Les Miserables*, and it became our go-to elixir when we needed to be healed by laughter. I still listen to it, and it still cracks me up. I can't describe it... just YouTube it; trust me.

March 2018 (age 15)

Snow

L Grey

March 4, 2018 (age 15)

And so winter ticks on
Frigid, unforgiving
Enveloping trees in greyscale
I've slept through the dark days
But the nights drag on for months
I am hibernating

Incubating growth
From what I hear outside is uninhabitable
Though I don't know
The windowsills are cold
A labyrinth of blankets keeps me warm
Further I sink into the sweat covered sheets of an unmade bed
The weeks are freezing
I am still, I am unmoving

Entry 8 (last journal entry)

L Grey
March 5th, 2018 (age 15)

i havent been sleeping. the dark circles under my eyes take up my whole face.
i look like
something that died and came back. I've treated my body as nothing more than a living,
breathing pill case. i dont know why im writing this. i think maybe because im afraid i'll die, and nobody will know how bad it was at the end. i dont know. im tired. this is hell

---

"Hey, Mom, do you think any of the medication I am on might be making it hard for me to pee?"

I gave her the look that I had given her so many times before. It was the look that said, "What do you mean? And why are you just telling me this now?"

"I'm really having trouble peeing. Like I have to push on my bladder to get anything out, and then it's just a tiny bit, so all day long it feels like I have to pee, but I can't get it out. It's really uncomfortable, and yeah, probably not a good thing."

I called Dr. Lubenow and asked him to recheck the imaging from where the spinal leads were placed. He assured me the images were clean and that there was no way the leads could cause any nerve damage to her bladder. I called Dr. Gary to see if any of her medications could have this side effect. He said it was unlikely but that we should wean her off the one or two that may have even a remote possibility of interrupting normal bladder function. We did. It did not change anything.

L spent most of March going to urologists who performed a series of invasive tests to try to understand what was going on. The conclusion they drew was that her brain was not sending proper nerve signals to her bladder, and thus it was not contracting to allow her to pee. Of course, no one could tell us why or whether the function would ever come back; rather, they taught L to use a catheter.

Upon learning this, Dr. Lubenow determined it was time for the spinal cord stimulator to be removed. Even though the images showed that everything was properly in place, it could not be coincidence, and there must be something about the stimulator and the leads that was impinging on her bladder function. Since the stimulator was not helping her leg pain as it was supposed to, he wanted it out. I wanted it out too. But the thought of another surgery, the idea that the trauma to L's body could exacerbate her CRPS, was overwhelming. We were faced with an impossible decision: leave the stimulator as is and risk ongoing complications or remove it and risk more surgical trauma. L and I talked about it at length. It was her body, and it had been through hell. She needed to have a voice. She decided to proceed with the surgery.

March 29, 2018, would be L's final surgery. I know how anxious I was as I watched them prep her. I can only imagine the anxiety she must have felt. Mercifully, it was uneventful as surgeries go. Her CRPS did not spread further. Nor did her bladder ever regain its ability to contract on its own; L would spend the rest of her life inserting a catheter every time she needed to relieve herself.

No More (work in progress)
L Grey
March 31, 2018 (age 15)

My heart beats at the rate of God
My breath is red and frozen
No more, we beg
No more
Spring peaks its head out from around the corner
Growth on the horizon
Playing hide-and-seek with winter
The clouds mock us
They laugh in fear
Screaming about the shapes they are not
The sky is thick and looming
I can smell a migraine in the air
Thunder is last year's hit still stuck in my head
A never ending record
The sun is dead behind my eyes
Maybe a Chernobyl storm will melt our skin
Wash clean the baseless divinity
In rancid physicality
My New Years resolution is to scrub away
This spring I will become an entity
At first light
At first downpour
I will transcend

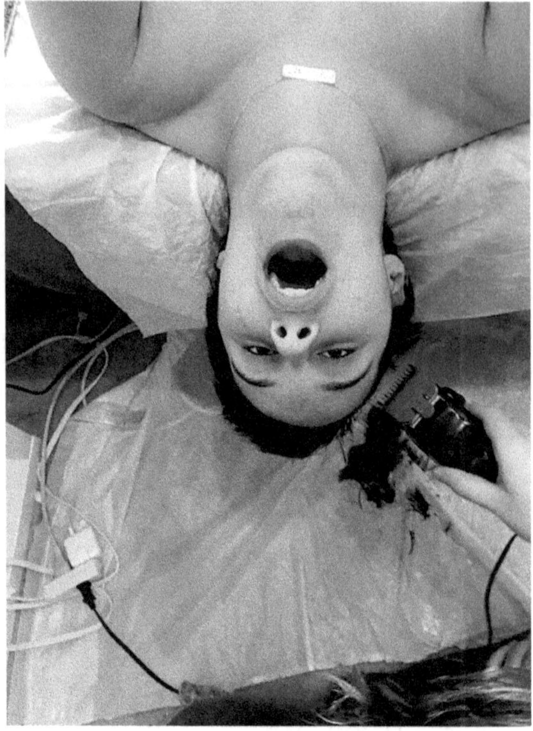

Wes shaving L's head, March 16, 2018, age 15.

L had been in bed for three months. The new spinal-cord stimulator had been removed, but nothing was getting better. Everything, it seemed, was getting worse. The pain was unrelenting, her heart rate rarely dipped below 170 at this point, and she had trouble taking full breaths. In addition to her shoulders dislocating daily, her hips now started to dislocate as well, no doubt a result of muscle deterioration from being bedridden. And her MCAS seemed to be accelerating. Her face would swell, and her lips would balloon to the point that they would start bleeding, the expansion pulling so hard on her thin skin that her lips would tear open. Dr. Gary started her on a new medication, cromolyn sodium (a mast-cell stabilizer), which L would need to take four times a day to try to manage her increasingly random allergic reactions. We also found a wonderful orthopedic doctor who fitted L for a hip brace, a medieval looking contraption that helped to keep her hips in their sockets while she slept. It felt like we were rowing hard upstream just to keep from drowning.

On Yiddish (work in progress)
L Grey
April 10, 2018 (age 15)

Yiddish is a language of tears
Every letter, every word, every poem
Is someone gone
They say that Jewish art
Jewish beauty
Is drawn in blood
That every Yiddish lullaby is an ode to what we have lost
Every Jewish metaphor is a story of sorrow
Each happy sounding klezmer beat
Is written in a minor key
I am the product of living
Of fruitless fighting
And holding on
Praying for another day
I am the product of tragic nostalgia
Heartbreaking kitsch
Loss and birth and everything unspoken
I am the product of swallowing your story so they cannot erase it
So that when they cut you open to harvest your identity
It is already digested and dispersed
So they cannot steal what we stood for
When they do an autopsy
My poems are written in English
But my story is written in endurance
It is spinning the world into something pretty
Something pithy

Yiddish is written in survival
Each letter is a battle cry
Each word is a tapestry
I am made of the language of living
Like my grandmother before me
And her mother before her

Atropos (The Riot)
L Grey
April 16, 2018 (age 15)

L'chaim
To death, and all things tragic
Cheers to Atropos
Who cuts the thread
To the alleyways and back rooms
Where we meet her again
I raise my glass to the cruelty
That outwits fate
A toast to the protests
All the things we fought for
For to every unmarked grave
To every one unmourned
Cheers to the standing
Who carry the caskets
Who hold the weight
Of bereavement
And weave the grief
Into uproar
A quiet, rotten toothed, swollen faced, shaky breathed, whispered;
"L'chaim-
To the riot"

May 11, 2018 (age 15)

"Okay, I have an idea... hear me out." She had clearly been researching something, getting all her ducks in a row.

"Can you talk to Dr. Gary about a port, you know, like a central line so that I could get a straight shot of saline directly into my bloodstream?" Before I could respond, she continued.

"It's not like I want any more things implanted in my body, but here's the thing. You know how fluids are supposed to be the best thing to regulate heart rate and blood pressure?"

"Yeah," I said. "I can't say I fully understand why, but I know that's what the doctors have told us."

"Well, the reason fluids help is because when you're dehydrated your blood thickens and your heart has to work harder to pump it, thus increasing your heart rate. Plus, dehydration diminishes your blood volume, so there literally isn't as much blood moving through your veins... and there you have it, folks, low blood pressure! But that's really not the point at the moment." She was on a roll. "The point is, no matter how much water and Gatorade I take in, it doesn't change my heart rate or blood pressure, but the times I've been in the hospital with IV saline, it's helped a lot. So, here's what I figure. My body is all kinds of fucked up. So, I think I'm not absorbing hydration from the fluids I drink, for whatever reason. But I think I can absorb it through IV. So, what if I got a port, and then I could have saline whenever I need it? If I could get my heart rate and blood pressure under control, maybe I'd have more energy for PT and life in general. You with me, Mom? You picking up what I'm puttin' down? You catching my drift? You feelin' it, Mr. Krabs?"

It made sense to me. I reached out to Dr. Gary, and he agreed that saline would be the best thing for her. He just didn't love the idea of her going through another procedure to get a port placed. And running a temporary IV through her arm that would need to be changed with every infusion didn't sound great either. But he liked the idea of IV saline. It was a Friday, and he wanted to think about it over the weekend to determine the least cumbersome way to go about it. Jessica, L's pediatrician, agreed.

May 13, 2018 (Mother's Day) 2:43 am (age 15)

Could you come in?

L was white as a ghost. "I can't get my heart rate down. It's never been this bad. I've been drinking Gatorade and water, but it's not helping, and it's really bad." She was short of breath and trying desperately to take a long, slow drag of air. I climbed in bed next to her and started telling her stories like I did when she was a little girl, hoping her heart would settle, even just a little. After about a half hour, she was getting annoyed by my presence and asked me to leave her room, assuring me she'd be okay. I gave her a kiss and walked out, pulling the door closed behind me (the way she liked it), but before it clicked shut, I turned and walked back in. Something told me she should not be alone, no matter how much she wanted to be.

"I'm sorry, honey, I know you want to be alone, but I just don't think you should be right now. I'll stay on the floor, but I need to be in here with you."

She didn't argue. We were both quiet in her dark room for about a minute, and then I heard thrashing. I stood up from the floor and saw L had tipped and was now face down, seizing violently. I quickly turned her head to the side, squeezed her hand, and rubbed her back, talking to her in the most measured, reassuring voice I could muster, not knowing if she could hear me but hoping that, subconsciously, the sound of my voice would guide her out of the seizure. She came out of it about a minute later, gasping violently for breath, as if she had been under water the whole time. "I peed," she whispered, recognizing that the only thing that got her to pee without a catheter was a seizure.

I knew we had to go to the hospital, but we sat quietly in her room for a few minutes so she could catch her breath first. She was disoriented as it was, and the trip to the hospital was going to be extraordinarily painful. She needed to just breathe for a minute. When she seemed to be strong enough, we made our way out of the house and to the ER. They immediately started her on a saline drip, and within minutes the color returned to her face, her heart rate improved (to about 120), and her blood pressure came back to a normal range. As it did, she became increasingly more alert and chatty, asking me to bring her latex gloves so she could blow them up and make them look like rooster feathers.

I told the ER doctors about her previous seizure almost a year earlier and how all of the EEGs came out normal, leaving us to believe it was a reaction to medication. They did another EEG, which also showed nothing abnormal. As they were shuffling in and out trying to figure out what to do, I had an "I should've had a V8!" moment. I noticed how quickly L's heart rate and blood pressure were regulated when they started the saline, and I began to wonder if her elevated heart rate and low blood pressure could have, in fact, caused the seizure in the first place. I began Googling. I quickly came across

"convulsive syncope." Essentially, if your heart is racing so violently out of control, your body can literally shut down—a fainting spell that looks like a seizure—so that it can reset itself. This made intuitive sense to me. When the doctor came back in the room, I asked if he thought that could be a possibility. "Let's give her more saline and see how she does."

By the time the second liter of saline was making its way through her body, it was a reasonable time in the morning to call Dr. Gary. I explained what had happened and also asked about convulsive syncope. He was right there with me. "Our girl," he laughed. "She's determined to get that port. She's not going to let us dawdle on this decision. We're going to arrange home health care. We are going to start with a regular IV in her arm to see how it works and how long the effects last before we schedule the placement of the port. We want to be sure before we do any more procedures." We left the hospital at 9:30 on Mother's Day morning exhausted but with L's heart at a manageable rate and the promise of a plan that might bring her more ongoing relief, at least from that particular symptom.

Later that afternoon, L gave me a Mother's Day present. It was a silver ring with her birthstone resting beside Jaz's birthstone, along with this note:

Momma,

Ok, first of all, let's get the unceremonious bullshit over with real quick - a little forest nymph snuck $60 into your gift bag to cover the cost of the gift itself, which I bought on your credit card, and assorted Lush products. You have to accept it, those are my Mother's Day rules. No takesies-backsies.

Alright, onto the fun stuff...

I'm not really sure where to start with the praise. You have done so much for me and Jaz, sacrificed so much more than I could ever hope to repay. You have given us more love than most people receive in a lifetime. It does not go unnoticed- by anybody. Me, Jaz, my friends, everybody with a human brain sees you as a superhero. You are the mother every woman aspires to be. You have led by example and shown me how to be a good person. You have taught me how to be kind, empathetic, independent, and mature. You are an absolute force to be reckoned with.

I know you are impossibly hard on yourself; I also know nothing I can ever say will change that. Nonetheless, I wish you'd cut yourself some slack. "Amazing" is far too weak of a word to describe you. I am forever grateful to have you as a mom. I am forever grateful to have you in my life. You bore me, brought me into the world, and have since worked nonstop to protect me from its dangers. You're the reason I'm here, and, like everything else, that is not something I will ever be able to repay. Thank you.

I love you. More than you know, more than I think I'll ever be able to articulate. You deserve the world and all the good things in it. I am better for knowing you.

Happy, happy Mother's day

-L

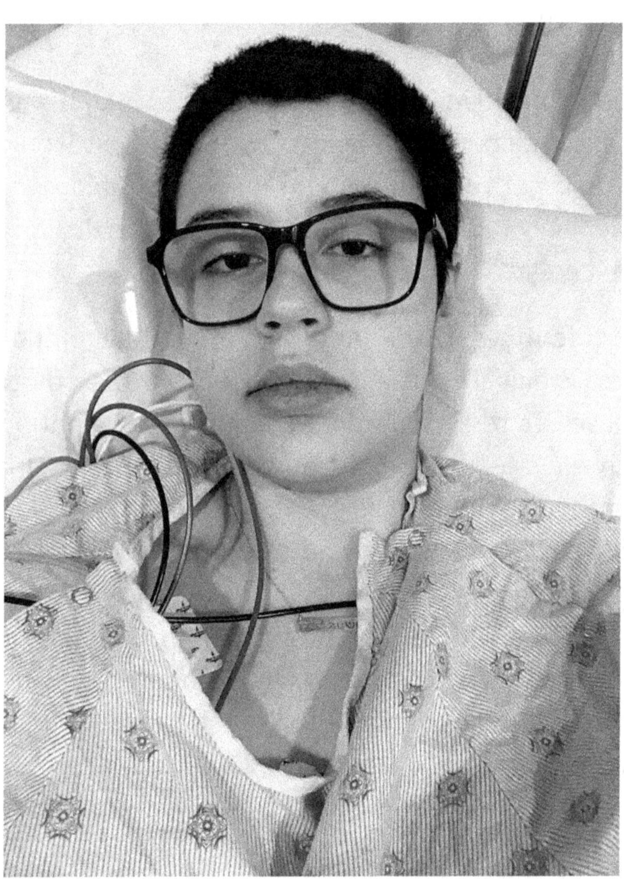

L in the hospital on Mother's Day morning.

May 23, 2018 (age 15)

The autoimmune hypothesis was growing in strength for both me and Dr. Gary. A few weeks prior he'd decided to have L take a test that was designed to diagnose PANDAS (pediatric autoimmune neuropsychiatric disorders associated with streptococcal infections). PANDAS is a neurological autoimmune disorder triggered by strep throat. We knew L did not have PANDAS, as her symptoms were totally different, but it fell within a broader category of autoimmune encephalopathy, which essentially is an inflammation of the brain. Since there were no other commercially available tests to look for autoimmune encephalopathy antibodies, the thinking went like this: If L tested positive, we would know for sure that she had autoimmune encephalopathy; if she tested negative, it wouldn't tell us much. It would not rule out autoimmune encephalopathy, it would just rule out encephalopathy caused by the particular antibodies that this test could detect.

The test identifies five neurologic autoimmune antibodies. If any one of them is elevated, it indicates significant neurologic autoimmune disease. L's results were in. Four of the five antibodies were significantly elevated. L's entire nervous system was being attacked by her own body—the war on her central nervous system causing the unyielding pain, and the war on her autonomic nervous system likely causing her other organ systems to shut down or run rampantly out of control. It was a moment of triumph and despair. Knowing that there was a root cause was strangely calming, and certainly validating, but the definitive knowledge that L had been fighting something that she was never going to beat with physical therapy alone was heartbreaking. And the prospects for treatment were limited and uncertain at best.

"What are the treatment options?" I asked Dr. Gary, knowing that I'd need to have these answers before talking to L.

"We're looking at two things. IVIG (intravenous immunoglobulin) and/or plasma exchange therapy. These are both messy, not likely to be covered by insurance, and have no guarantees, so you need to think about what you want to do."

"Which do we do first, and how quickly can we start?"

"I had a feeling you'd say that. We'll start with IVIG; it is far less invasive than plasma exchange. She'll need an infusion anywhere from once a week to once a month, totaling no more than two grams of IVIG per kilogram of body weight over the course of the month. The exact frequency and amount will be determined by what she can tolerate. We'll start slow and titrate up. She will likely feel worse before she feels better, and it could be months before she feels any relief. This is colossally expensive, so we are going to try to get insurance to cover it. It will take a few weeks to sift through that, so sit tight. I know you're eager, but you've waited this long, and I don't want this to bankrupt you. In the meantime, let's get the IV saline going and see how she does on that."

I went into L's room and shared the test results with her.

"Halle-fuckin-lujah! I'm not crazy! All those idiots who said I was making this up...I feel so validated!" She clearly felt satisfied in knowing what was behind all of this. "Let me guess, the options are IVIG or plasma exchange. My vote, if I get a vote, is IVIG as a start. Plasma exchange sounds barbaric, like old-world leeching."

"That's what Dr. Gary and I were thinking," I said.

"Cool. But, Mom, it's a fortune. I know that. I've looked this shit up. I'm worried you're never going to be able to retire. I know you're the sole breadwinner, and I don't want you killing yourself at work. I see how much you shoulder, how hard you work to support us. And even though you don't complain, I know it takes a toll."

"Stop worrying about me. Not your job. Besides, what do you think I'm going to be doing, sitting at a beach in Hawaii with you next to me in a hospital bed, unable to move, while I'm enjoying a Pina Colada?"

"Touché."

In retrospect, I think the confirmation that her nervous system was under attack gave L something she had always sought and coveted—*truth*. When I think about it, it's what drove L in life and what she has been determined to help us all see in her death. It's what she has always craved, searched for, fought for, and stood for. It is why she was determined to document her journey, her pain, and her courage. It is why she started a podcast and became a champion for anyone and everyone who had ever been marginalized. It is why she had an insatiable curiosity and quest for knowledge. It is why she was emphatic about getting her story out there and why she is guiding my hand at this moment. L was, and is, a warrior for truth. She hungered to not only honor her own truth but to help others find freedom in knowing theirs. And in seeing the unequivocal test results, she finally had confirmation. She finally had truth. I see now that this gave her the peace of mind, two months later, to realize the fate that she understood so many years before and to emancipate her soul from her body.

June 2018 (age 15)

L started getting IV saline at home through a regular line in her arm. The nurse would come, hook her up with a liter, and be on her way. It was a successful test in that we learned that saline worked for a short time. Each liter would give her about eight hours of a better-regulated heart rate. The problem was she could only receive saline this way two, maybe three times a week. L had horribly weak veins, and even the skilled nurse had trouble finding them, and often her vein would collapse before the full liter made its way into her body. With each blown vein, the options were narrowing, and soon she wouldn't be able to have an IV in her arm at all. Dr. Gary agreed it was time for the port. It was successfully placed on June 22nd, and for the first time in years, she could stay hydrated. L was meticulous about following the nurse's protocol to a T in order to keep the port completely sterile. She was not going to let herself fall victim to infection. She was not going to fall prey to a foreign attack, and she was not going to leave this world on anyone's terms but her own.

In the background, several things were happening. We were consulting with several neurologists who agreed with the IVIG recommendation, and we were working on insurance to approve it. We were discovering that on top of all of this, L may have had an underlying chronic Lyme disease.

L had been tested for Lyme when her illness first began, and the results were negative. We were urged to have her retested with a more sophisticated and sensitive test, and the new results showed positive for Lyme bacteria. Dr. Gary was not happy. "Lyme complicates everything. It's controversial, and there are a million schools of thought about it, but we can't ignore it." In a way, it made sense. It was possible that an undetected and untreated Lyme disease could have triggered an autoimmune response, which then took on a life of its own. So, even though the autoimmune disease was an issue unto itself, if L did have Lyme, that would need to be treated as well. Treating one without the other wouldn't get us very far. We consulted with infectious disease experts, and everyone landed in the same place. Since L had a port anyway, she should start on a round of IV Rocephin, a powerful antibiotic known to combat Lyme. If L did not have Lyme, it would do no harm, but if she did, it would help kill it. This decision was not an easy one. There are Lyme specialists who insist antibiotics make it worse. There is more inconclusive research than definitive answers, and the experts in the field do not unanimously agree. But Rocephin was a standard, well-known, and well-regarded treatment, and no one we talked to had opposition.

"This changes our timeline a little," Dr. Gary said. "I want her on Rocephin for at least a month before we start IVIG. If she does have Lyme, we need to get that under control before starting the IVIG. A month won't kill it completely (it could take months or years), but it should at least make a dent, and we need to make a dent before going for the IVIG. We're still waiting on insurance anyway... what do you think?"

We didn't love it, but then again, we didn't love any of our options.

Jaz was away at camp while all this was going on, and L was clearly missing her, never abandoning her role as protective big sister. She sent Jaz a series of bunk-note emails over the summer, trying to make Jaz smile, trying to hide her pain from Jaz, and, in retrospect, leaving her sister love letters that she could carry with her forever, L's personality jumping off the pages.

June 21, 2018 (age 15)

Subject: *Jazzzzz what's good yo it's L*

Hey you. This here is a photo of Sappho- she's an ancient greek poet who wrote almost exclusively about loving women. She lived on the island of Lesbos, and that's where the word lesbian comes from. How're you holding up? I miss you- the house is too quiet without your sass and hot takes. I hope you're having a ball, and if you're not, know that I am sending you tremendous amounts of love and good vibes. Gonna get a port tomorrow, so woo hoo for fun drugs! I'll update you after the surgery, but it's a super minor little thing.

Love you, L

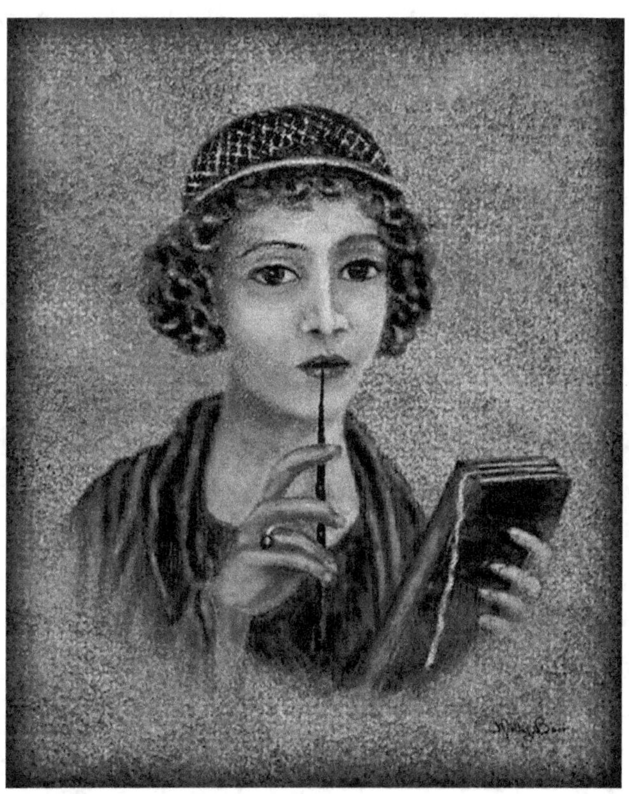

June 25, 2018 (age 15)

Subject: *Read this it's important and full of love - from L*

Hey Plumhead, How're you holding up? I miss you a lot- like, way more than I thought I would. Your presence just makes the house feel warmer. I feel slightly empty not talking to you every day! Also, just so you know, the port surgery went great! No pain at all and everything is healing nicely. I want you to know that I am so incredibly proud and honored to be your sister. It's not lost on me how much you have gone through this year. Healing can be so exhausting and brutal, but I've watched you endure and conquer so much. You are a beautiful, intelligent, witty, loving, amazing person and I hope you know how much you mean to me. I love you beyond what I can try and fit into a bunknote. ANYWAY, enough of that fucking sappy shit. Did you know Sperm Whales are called Sperm Whales because the guy who discovered them thought that the fluid surrounding their brain was sperm? Also did you know the Tampon was invented to absorb blood from battle wounds in WWI? I just learned that one today. Take care of yourself, know that I love you and I'm thinking about you and I miss you!

L

July 3, 2018 (age 15)

Subject: *Rasputin*

I feel so bad for whoever is in the camp office printing up pictures of random historical figures. They probably think I'm nutso, which, I mean, to be fair...Anyway this creepy motherfucker is Rasputin. He was a Russian peasant who slept with the Russian queen. He was a "mystic" and tried to cure the queen's son of hemophilia (a blood disease, but this was like 1900 and it was Russia so, you know, mysticism instead of medicine.) Also people tried to assassinate him like 6 times and he lived through poison and like 8 gunshot wounds. The closest we've ever gotten to a real life wizard, and he was a Russian peasant having an affair with a monarch. Go figure. Oh, and there's a kitschy 80s song about him. It's a real bop, too. I love you, I miss you, I hope you are enjoying your random historical figures. Have an amazing 4th of July. And write me a letter smh. Or send dirt. Whatever floats your boat.

Love you, your favorite sibling

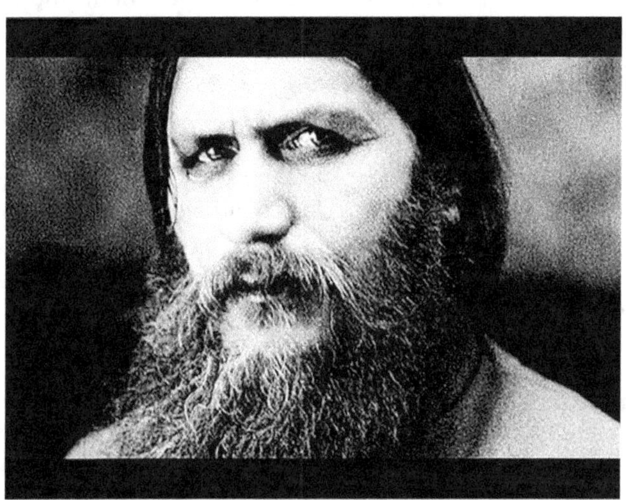

July 7, 2018 (age 15)

L had started the Rocephin a few days prior, and other than a little diarrhea, she seemed to be tolerating it without much of an issue. But on July 7 she became violently nauseous, retching with even the smallest sip of water. I asked Dr. Gary if this could be a side effect from the Rocephin, since antibiotics often messed with L's stomach. "It's possible," he said, "but unlikely. The benefit of IV antibiotic is that they tend to be much easier on the stomach than oral antibiotics. Let's discontinue the Rocephin for a day or two and see if she feels better."

We stopped the Rocephin, hoping the nausea would pass. Instead, it got worse.

July 8, 2018, 1:00 am (age 15)

Subject: *I planted Bob!*

Guess what? Bob Ross is officially planted! Finally! It's 1am as I'm writing this and I couldn't sleep, so I thought "what better use of my insomnia than to curate my chia pet?" I'm hoping he'll start sprouting before you get home!! I also got your birthday gift in the mail today! I didn't know what you wanted but I think you'll like it! I hear you have a concussion. That sucks ass. Just super unlucky. Although sort of badass, in like an absurd kinda way. I hope you feel as well as you possibly can. Rest, sleep, take care of yourself. If I was there I'd offer you my preemo migraine meds. I'm thinking about you a lot these days. I miss you a lot. Maybe when you get back you can do my makeup or something. Maybe a Starbucks extravaganza? Remember that guy in Starbucks who brought in his own fully cooked meal? Priceless. I love you, have fun, be well. Wes says hi, by the way. I told him I'd pass that along to you

<3 L

July 8, 2018 (age 15)

8:29 pm (text)

Hey doesn't really matter but fyi threw the rice and remaining toast up

July 12, 2018 (age 15) (Jaz's 14th birthday)

3:12 pm (text)

You don't have to come in but I just want to let you know that I just threw up some of a bagel that I ate like 25 hours ago.

She clearly was not digesting anything that went into her body.

6:29 pm (text)

Can you come in I want to show you something

I walked into L's room, and she was lying on her back. Her stomach looked like she was six months pregnant, swollen beyond recognition, despite her inability to keep any food down for the past five days. L was hydrated from the saline, but she had taken in no calories and was incredibly weak. "This is not from the antibiotic. You need to take her into the ER," Dr. Gary told me.

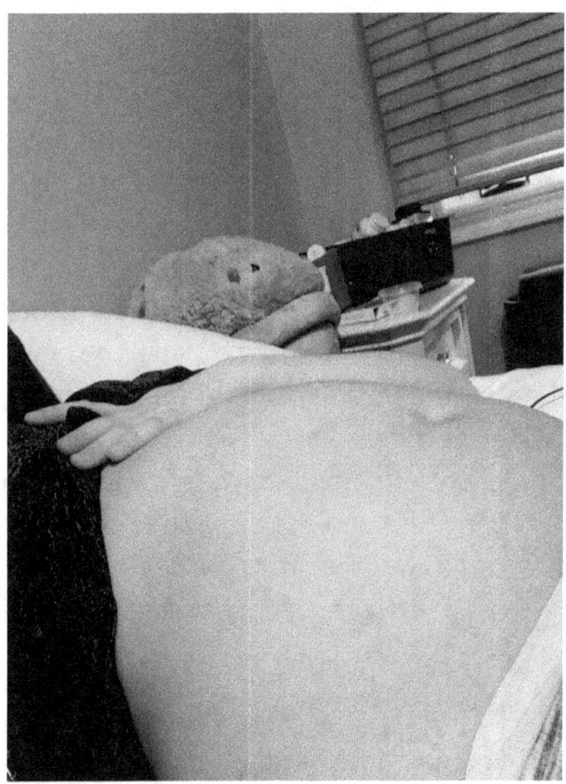

L's stomach after not eating for five days, July 12, 2018, age 15.

July 13–17, 2018 (age 15)

We were back at Lurie Children's Hospital, where they put her on dextrose so she could at least have calories and were running myriad tests and swallow studies to confirm what we suspected. L had gastroparesis, which basically means the muscles that are supposed to automatically push food through your digestive system weren't doing their job. So, L would take a bite of food and it would just sit there, unable to work its way through her body, and eventually it would just come back up undigested. The good news is, there are medications to manage it, and L seemed to respond after a few days. The bad news, of course, is that no one knew why it happened, nor could they guarantee that it wouldn't happen again.

I did my best to try to stay calm and positive around L, but we both knew what the other was thinking. Was this a random bout of gastroparesis? Or was this one more major organ system shutting down, under attack by her own immune system? The doctors there didn't even attempt to answer this question. By their own admission, they were focused on getting her to tolerate food. Any larger, systemic issue would need to be handled by her primary physicians. L and I pretended to be in the present moment. We pretended to be focused on her regaining her appetite and keeping food down. But hammering through both our minds was the unspoken question of what this really meant. I knew, without a doubt, that if her digestive system was shutting down, that if she could not eat, she would no longer have the will to live.

At some point during those five days in the hospital, I went over to my aunt's house two blocks away to shower. My dad and sister were with L, and the two-block walk in the open air was cruelly short. The door to my aunt's apartment was unlocked, and I walked into her outstretched arms. Her son had drowned two years prior, and she knew my fear. I fell into her arms and cried heavy, uncontrollable sobs. She held me close, knowing that there was nothing either of us could say.

L and I returned home on July 17th, her digestion temporarily restored. Waiting for her was a box of 120 pouches of oyster crackers, compliments of her grandparents.

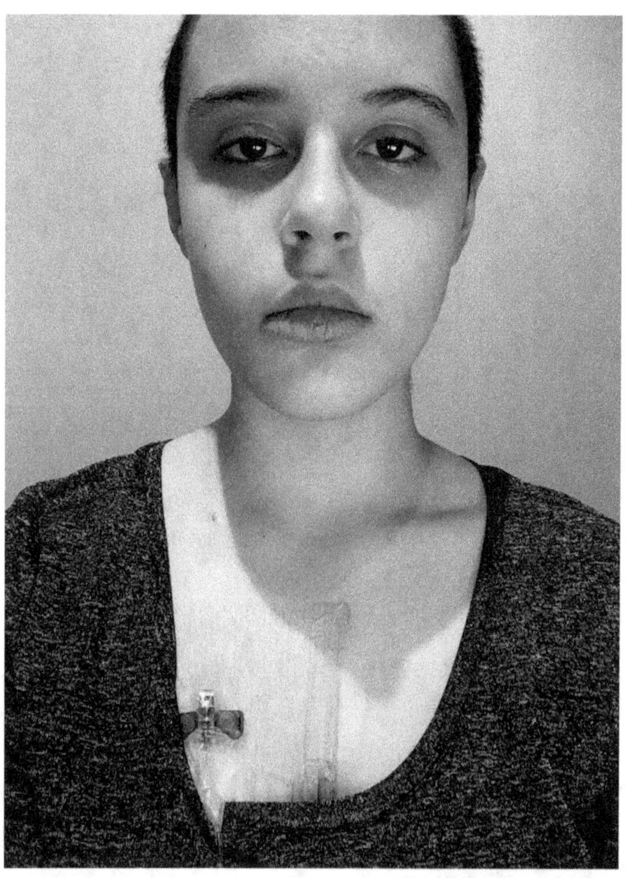

L's final selfie, July 2018, age 15. When I look at her eyes,
it is as if she is begging to be freed.

July 20, 2018 (age 15)

8:41 pm (text)

Could I borrow your phone and laptop for like 3 minutes? I'm voting for myself in a writing contest but I need to do it on different devices

July 21, 2018 (age 15, the day before she died)

2:13 am

Will you come in?

L was lying down, her feet dangling over the side of her bed, dripping pools of blood. On the floor were towels, soaked with blood. Every single one of her scars from her lesions had opened simultaneously, with new lesions emerging on top of them. She had 40 open wounds on her feet, each raw and angry and bleeding uncontrollably. I took her hand and squeezed it tightly, planting a kiss on her cheek. We quietly went about cleaning each lesion, applying antibiotic ointment, and carefully wrapping her feet in gauze until it looked like her feet were wearing boxing gloves. Neither of us was able to find many words, so we sat close in quiet company, exchanging I-love-yous while we alternated in and out of fitful sleep until the sun came up. After that, she wanted to be alone.

6:43 pm (later that day)

"I think I'm ready to be published," L declared. "All the poems I've been working on and the short stories I've written... I've organized them into a book, and I want to get it published. To be honest, it's more like a need—I *need* to get it published. You know, it's part of my whole arrogant legacy/god-complex thing. I have this irrational need to have an impact on the world. You feel me? Will you help me get it published?" "Of course, sweetheart," I paused, "I'm proud of you." "Cool," she said.

"Oh, and I know what I want to do for my 16th birthday. I want a big, blowout sweet 16," she laughed, "which, you know, means me and about four friends having burgers, fries, and milkshakes at DMK!" "Sounds great!" I said.

"You have to promise."

"Of course, honey," I said. "You know we can do whatever you want to celebrate."

She held out her hand. "Deal?" she asked.

"Deal." We shook on it so that it was binding.

"Can I order a Domino's pizza?

"Do you think your stomach can handle it?"

"I'm really craving something with flavor, you know. I do love me my oyster crackers, but I need some sauce. The worst that happens is I throw it up."

Her pizza arrived, and I brought it up to her room. I plopped myself down in her wheelchair by her bed, as I often did to keep her company. She let me linger for a bit and then asked if I wouldn't mind leaving her alone. "I just need a Zen moment with my pizza." She put her hands in a prayer position, closed her eyes, and breathed in the aroma of sauce and cheese. "I understand. I love you, sweetheart. I'll come back later to give you your meds."

"Oh, and one more thing," she said, "my phone is acting kind of funky, so if you call or text and I don't answer right away, don't freak out, okay?"

"Got it, thanks for letting me know. I'll take it to the Apple store tomorrow.

I came back in around 11:30 that night to dole out her meds. It was clear she was not in the mood for company. I gave her a hug and a kiss on the head. She held out her hand and gave me a fist bump.

"I love you more than anything, sweet girl. Call me if you need me."

"I will. I love you too. Good night, Momma."

July 22, 2018 (age 15)

I woke up with a pounding headache, the thunderstorm in my mind posing a stark contrast to the warm summer sun outside. I had fallen into a restless sleep at around 3:00am, after repeatedly peeking in on L. I needed something to clear my head. It was a Sunday, and with no physical therapy to wake up for, L would sleep until at least 2:00. With Mia home and on watch, Jaz and I headed to an 11:45 am Soul Cycle class. I'm not one who typically enjoys classes; I usually prefer the solitude of a walk or run to the company of others, but Jaz introduced me to Soul Cycle, and we were both hooked. There was something about riding to the rhythm of the music in a dark room that was, in fact, soothing to the soul. And there was something about Dylan, our favorite instructor; he could tap into the depths of my experience without even knowing it with the playlists he would choose for class. In the studio I could lose myself for 45 minutes, and it had become something that Jaz and I loved doing together.

Jaz and I clipped in and let the music carry us; the last song Dylan played was Fleetwood Mac's "The Chain," and by the time it was over, my headache was gone, replaced with Stevie's mystical voice seeming to swallow me… *We will never break the chain*… ringing in my ears over and over. I texted L to let her know we were going to run an errand. I didn't expect her to respond; it was slightly after noon, and history would suggest she'd be asleep for two more hours.

Jaz needed shoes, so we made a quick stop at Nordstrom. I texted L again and noticed that my previous text was green, instead of blue, which usually suggests a phone in airplane mode or somehow not connected to Wi-Fi. The reception in Nordstrom was notoriously spotty, and L had told me her phone had been acting up, but I did find it curious. When Jaz and I got into the car, I called L and left her a voicemail. I couldn't put my finger on it, but something was off. Jaz and I drove home in relative silence, the anxiety in both of us quietly building.

We got home, and Jaz went into her room to rest and listen to music. I decided to check on L. I turned the knob on her door slowly, to try to be as quiet as a I could, and I peeked in. The blinds on the windows were drawn and it was dark in her room. From where I stood in the hallway, I could make out her shape under the blankets on her bed, but something didn't look right. It wasn't immediately clear. It took me a second to put it together. Her wheelchair wasn't next to her bed.

I had just come from my bedroom, and she wasn't in there, and the stairlift was parked upstairs, so she could not be downstairs. She could barely get out of bed, let alone leave the house. There was nowhere she could have gone. These thoughts entered my mind opaquely. I was not consciously piecing things together; rather, I was taking stock at a subconscious, blurry level. I walked into her room, still only half registering that her wheelchair was nowhere to be seen, and I went over to her bed. I gently peeled back a blanket to give her a kiss. She wasn't there. In her place, she had piled pillows to give the illusion that she was in bed. Everything was still blurry. Anxiety and fear took hold, but nothing had crystallized yet. "Where was she?" Her bathroom door was closed, and there was no light coming through the bottom, but I made my way toward the door anyway. I walked into her dark bathroom and saw the silhouette of her wheelchair next to the bathtub, but still no L. I flicked on the light.

L was in the bathtub, her head resting gently on the tile wall. Her right hand was holding Grazer and her left hand was on her stomach.

Her lips were ever so slightly blue, and a small trickle of blood crept from her nose and her mouth. The water in the tub was red, stained with the blood from her open lesions.

"L!" I screamed, "L, L, L." I cradled her cool head in my hands, still not sure what exactly had happened, not knowing if she had hit her head, had a seizure, or made her own decision to end her pain. None of that was registering. The only thought racing through my head was "Oh, my God. Today is the day. Today is the day."

"Mia!" I screamed, "Mia!" I ran into Jaz's room. "Go get Mia. Now. And don't come into L's room." I raced back into L's room, frantically looking for my phone to call 911. Mia was there in seconds; she had already called 911 and was on the phone with the paramedics who were on their way. I was in the bathtub with L, holding her head, her hands, trying to give her CPR even though I could tell from the coldness of her skin that it was far too late.

"She's gone, Mia. I know it. She's dead," I kept crying over and over.

Mia looked shocked, "No, no, no, she can't be. We have to get her out of the water, then she'll be okay."

We lifted her out of the tub and settled her onto the floor, screaming her name and willing her to breathe. Out of the corner of my eye, I saw an empty pill bottle on the floor and a notebook page with her handwriting. I thought I saw the word "rainbow" and the phrase "I love you momma," but I couldn't be sure. There must have been sirens in the background, but I heard nothing other than my own breathing as I willed my breath to become hers. The paramedics were there in an instant.

"No pulse," the arriving paramedic said to someone. I felt another person's arms around me. A woman dressed in police clothes. "You need to leave the room, sweetheart. We'll let you know everything that is going on, but you can't stay in here." She ushered me out to the hallway where I sat on the chest outside L's room that housed our ski clothes. She sat next to me, holding my hand. Mia was there on my other side.

"We have to take care of Jaz. Mia, where is Jaz? I need you to find her and make sure she's okay."

I don't know how Mia did what she did in those moments. Mia was a second mom to L, and somehow, through her own shock and grief, she had the wherewithal to find Jaz and comfort her, and to call everyone she needed to call. Later that night, I learned that, upon hearing my screams, Jaz had immediately grabbed her phone and run out to the driveway to await the paramedics. She called her grandparents. They were at the house within 30 seconds, arriving just as the paramedics were. Among the many things I would come to be grateful for was knowing that Jaz was not alone in those moments.

But as I sat on the chest outside L's room, I knew none of this. I just knew that L was gone, and I didn't know what to do. "She's gone," I said to the police officer sitting next to me. "She's gone. I know she's gone. Please just tell me."

"She's gone," she whispered to me as my body heaved.

A slow stream of people started to make their way upstairs to me. First, L's grandma, who had been with Jaz on the driveway. I remember the vibrant salmon color of her shirt that I clawed as we cried. Then Marcy, Jaz's therapist, who arrived that afternoon and stayed all week. She held me close as I cried. Then my dad, whose sobs echoed mine. "What am I going to do? What am I going to do?" I pleaded with him. "I don't know," he croaked. "I don't know."

At some point, someone told me I needed to go downstairs. My clothes were still damp and stained pink with blood, but I didn't want to change. The scene in my kitchen was surreal; familiar faces of parents, aunts, uncles, and friends, contorted in unfamiliar forms; a sea of tears pierced by gut-wrenching sobs. Everyone's red eyes turned to me, and I saw arms reaching for hugs, but I blew past them, unable to look directly at anyone. "Where's Jaz?" was all I could say. "I need to find Jaz." The swarm of people seemed to part, and there she was. I ran to her, and we hugged as if our next breath depended on it. I quickly whisked her into the downstairs bedroom, away from the crowds, where we lay on the bed, crying in each other's arms. I have no idea how long we were there.

"Will we be okay?" she asked. "Will we ever be okay? Will we ever be happy again?"

"We're going to be more than okay. We already are. We have the best guardian angel looking out for us. I promise you, Jazzy, we are going to be happy again. L is going to help us."

Over the next few hours, the house seemed to swell with people. I was glad they could comfort each other, but I wanted no part of it. I just wanted to be with L. The paramedics assured me they would not remove her body from the house before letting me see her. The police commissioner, Gerry, stayed by my side, explaining everything that would happen over the next few days, then re-explaining when I couldn't recall it. He told me what the coroner would do and explained that there was a note, which the police needed but that I would get back the next day. He promised. He told me we'd all be able to see her again at the funeral home. When the police and paramedics had done all they could do and it was time for them to go, he asked if I really wanted to see L before they took her out of the house. "She'll look better at the funeral home once they've had a chance to clean her up. Are you sure you don't want to wait for that?"

"I need to see her now, Gerry, please."

"Okay."

He took my hand and helped me walk up the stairs to her room. She was on the floor of her bedroom, her body encased in an orange plastic bag with a zipper down the middle, leaving only her face exposed.

I knelt beside her and kissed her cool forehead, running her fuzzy buzzed hair through my fingers. I took my thumb and smoothed her eyebrows. When she was a baby and she would fight to keep her eyes open as the heaviness of sleep fell upon her, I would smooth her eyebrows, and it seemed to be the last little push needed to get her to close her eyes all the way and fully fall asleep. I smoothed them just that way. I kissed her swollen lips a dozen times. I nuzzled into her neck and breathed in deeply so that the scent of her could linger in my nostrils forever. And then I sang to her our lullaby.

Time to go to sleep, my sweet baby girl, it is now time to close your eyes and go to sleep.

I'll be right here in the morning when you wake up, but now it is time to go to sleep.

I love you, my sweet baby girl.

Gerry took my hand and led me back downstairs. "I've been doing this for 40 years, and I've seen and heard a lot of things," he said, "but I've never seen anything like that. I will never forget listening to you sing to your daughter. You're going to be okay. She's going to make sure of it."

It was getting dark by the time the house started to empty, and Jaz was adamant that she did not want to sleep at home. We put on pajamas and decided to head to her grandparents' house. As we were about to leave, Mia walked over to me and handed me Grazer. "How did you get him?" I asked.

"They wouldn't let anyone in the bathroom."

"I just went in there and got him. I didn't care. I knew you needed him. He is all washed."

So, in the frenzy of all that was happening, Mia was quietly and lovingly washing and drying Grazer, knowing exactly the comfort that he would bring me that day, and every day since. "May I come with you tonight?" she asked. "Of course, you can. Of course, you can."

We got settled at Jaz's grandparents, Jaz and I in one room and Mia in the other. Jaz and I lay on the bed, holding each other and Grazer. She drifted in and out of sleep, while I lay awake listening to the steady rhythm of her breathing, inhaling her still-little-girl smell. Images of L filled my head, and in my ears I could still hear Stevie's voice... *We will never break the chain.*

PART III: AFTER

"You have to meet with Lisa Nitzkin," my friend Amy insisted.

"I'm going to make it happen for you. I'm going to introduce you." When I did finally meet Lisa two months later, we embraced like long lost sisters, though we had actually never laid eyes on each other. It felt, simultaneously, like love at first sight and as if we had known each other for a lifetime.

July 23–July 27, 2018

That week. It will forever be known as "that week." I had decided to hold her funeral service on Friday, July 27th, to allow for some of her friends to make it into town. That left us with four days of an impromptu Shiva. The formal Shiva would be on Friday after her service but informally, the house would fill with people around 11:00 am and wouldn't empty until late at night. People would come and go, planning for the actual Shiva on Friday, congregating in the kitchen and crying, a never-ending stream of food somehow materializing, despite my total lack of appetite. Parts of that week are a blur, but parts of it are more vivid and clear than at any other time of my life. What stood out the most was L.

July 23, 2018

When Jaz and I came home the morning after L's passing, Jaz was surprised at how calm she felt walking into the house. She thought she would be scared or anxious, but she wasn't. Home still felt like home. It still felt safe. She and I sat outside in the backyard while we still had the house to ourselves, and I let my gaze float up to the sky. I can remember the exact blue of the sky, the bright green of the leaves on the trees, and the way the sun danced with the morning fog, creating rays so tangible it felt like I could reach out and touch them. Soon, L's face filled the sky, smiling with a wisp-like body trailing behind. "There you are sweetheart," I said aloud. She started doing somersaults and twirling. I could see her flying through the air, diving into crystal water and coming back up, her smile having grown, the words "I'm free" booming through the sky.

Her pediatrician, Jessica, came by that morning before the house got too crowded. She sat with me in the morning sun.

"She took a bottle of Norco. She must have gotten it from the back of my medicine cabinet from one of her prior surgeries," I told her. "Would she have suffered? Would she have struggled or gagged, or felt anything scary?" "No," she assured me. "I'm not just saying this because I'm your friend. I'm telling you she went to sleep and didn't feel a thing. I promise you." "I need to tell you something else," she said. "You need to reframe your thinking, and you need to understand that your daughter had a terminal illness.

There was no cure. She was not going to get better, and she knew it. And no one can survive in that much pain forever. It's not survivable. Only she could determine when her body had gone as far as it could go. She made a sound decision, and she was of right mind. You need to think of this as euthanasia. Your daughter was extraordinarily brave."

We were both crying at this point. "I know. With every fiber of my being I know this. I might need you to remind me a thousand times that she did not suffer when she passed."

"I'll remind you a million times."

Later that afternoon Gerry came by, as promised, with L's phone, computer, and the note she wrote. Of everything L ever wrote, her note to me on July 22nd was, by far, the most beautiful. I'm choosing to keep most of it private, but I am sharing the last paragraph, as it foretells the magic and beauty that would unfold before me in every day since her passing.

I am in every raven and rainbow you see. We'll see each other again before you know it. It's time for me to sleep now. Goodnight, Mommy. It's time to say goodnight.

I love you Momma,

L

July 25, 2018

The memorial arrangements had been made, and it was time for us to go to the funeral home to say one last goodbye to L's physical body before she was cremated. Grandparents, aunts, and uncles would all meet us there. At first, I thought Jaz should stay home. I was worried that she would not be prepared to see her sister in death, and I did not want her to be haunted by images she couldn't shake. But Jaz wanted to come, and I could not deny her the opportunity to kiss her sister goodbye. We agreed that I would visit with L first, and if I thought it would not be too scary for Jaz, I would then bring her in.

When we arrived, the director ushered me into the sanctuary. L was beautiful and was resting peacefully. She was wearing her favorite knit beanie on her head, a shirt that read "fuck shit" with a heart and a skull and crossbones on it, super-soft pajama pants, and her patent leather Doc Martens. She was wrapped snuggly in her rainbow blanket, or "glaynket" as she called it (a combination of gay + blanket). After kissing her lips, cheeks, forehead, and hands, I unwrapped her blanket so that I could touch her legs. Her legs, which had been on fire for so long, were now cold to the touch. Her legs, which could not be touched for three-and-a-half years, now flopped gently to each side, the bulky Doc Martens highlighting how skinny her calves were. I massaged her cold legs with my warm hands, willing the heat from my body to transfer to her and warm her up. Still, cold as they were, I marveled that I could touch them without her flinching, without there being any pain.

I brought Jaz in, and she gently brushed her fingertips across L's cheek. "Hi, L. It's me." Jaz was not freaked out. She was not at all uncomfortable being with L's body. But she was very disturbed by the color of lipstick L was wearing. It was a mild, nude color, and Jaz was not having it.

"We have to change her lipstick," Jaz said. "This is so not her color. L would not be happy with this color. We need something dark and edgy and goth. We are not letting them take her until we get the color right."

I chuckled because Jaz was completely right. And she had become quite protective of her older sister. We rejoined the rest of the family in the waiting area, and while they each went in to have a private moment with L, we searched for the right shade of lipstick. My aunt had a good dark shade that she was happy to donate to the cause. Once everyone had had a chance to say goodbye to L, I took Jaz back in. What then transpired is something I will never forget. It was the most tender, loving exchange I had ever seen between my girls. Jaz took a piece of Kleenex and gently wiped away the neutral shade, talking to L the whole time, assuring her that she was going to get the right color on her, laughing at how clearly the funeral home workers didn't know who they were dealing with. She then started to apply a deep maroon to L's lips, looking at L's face from multiple angles to make sure it was evenly applied. She would lean in close, and then stand back, making corrections as she went. When she got some lipstick outside the lines, she licked her finger and rubbed away the smudge with her spit, the way a grandmother might. Jaz probably spent 10 minutes talking to her sister, applying her makeup so that it was just right, oblivious to everything else around her. Because L spent all of her adolescence sick, they did not have many opportunities to do girly, sisterly things. And yet here they were, in the last minutes that they would spend together in the flesh, doing their makeup as if it were the most natural thing in the world. I stayed back and remained quiet, not wanting to disturb them, a tear rolling down my cheek as a prideful smile spread across my face. When Jaz felt the lipstick was perfect, she did a little happy dance and then leaned over her sister, planting a soft kiss on her cool, maroon lips. "Good night, L. I love you."

July 27, 2018

Wes had arrived the night before, and I got up early to buy him his favorite Dunkin Donuts coffee with hazelnut creamer before heading to the synagogue for L's memorial service. When I got home with the coffee, my friend Cristina from New Jersey was in the kitchen with Wes, and two of L's other friends were there as well. We all hugged each other, and I excused myself to go upstairs to get myself and Jaz ready. Jaz looked older than she had just a week before, and I found her upstairs looking for the right pair of shoes to wear to the service.

"I have an idea," I said. "Give me one second."

I walked into L's closet and found a pair of LGBT Docs. They were black with rainbow-colored writing all over them. We had purchased them, with hope, the prior summer in Arizona, and they had sat in her closet unworn ever since.

"What do you think?" I asked Jaz.

"Perfect!" she exclaimed. They were two sizes too big for her little feet, but she didn't seem to care.

The service was mesmerizing. Hundreds of people, from every phase of our lives, poured into the synagogue. Just before the service began, a young woman with a shock of short blue hair and Elvis Costello glasses wheeled herself into the synagogue. I did a double take. She looked exactly like L. She was crying as she was trying to maneuver her wheelchair through the crowd.

"Who is this?" I wondered. I walked over to her and introduced myself. "I'm Ashton," she said. "I just learned of L's passing, and I've been traveling all night from Virginia to get here. There are dozens of L's friends who wanted to be here, but so many of us are disabled, and many of them couldn't physically get here. So, I am representing all of us. She has changed our lives. You need to know how much we love her."

I was stunned. I know how difficult and painful travel can be when you are in a wheelchair. I know how intimidating it must have been for her to wheel into the sanctuary amongst hundreds of mourners who couldn't help but look twice when they saw her. And, yet, there she was. I quickly found L's other friends who knew Ashton and made room for her to sit with them.

While I was still reeling from the shock of seeing L's lookalike, the rabbi motioned for everyone to take their seats, and he began the service. It opened with an acoustic version of "Don't Stop Believin,'" and it only took one note on the piano before the tears began flowing freely. I closed my eyes, held Jaz's hand, felt her lean her head into my neck, which became wet with her tears, and felt myself transported to the summer of 2010 when L performed her own rendition. The crowds around me faded away, and I became aware only of Jaz's warmth, the sound of the cantor's voice, the wetness on my cheeks, and the undeniable energy of L.

My dad, my sister, and Mia each delivered a beautiful eulogy. The cantor read the eulogy Jaz had prepared, along with several poems L wrote before she got sick. And then it was my turn. I made my way onto the bema, and with L by my side, I began.

My Sweet Baby Girl
Vanessa Lynn
July 27, 2018

L, when I told people I was going to speak today, they thought I was crazy, that it would be too hard, too painful. But how could I not? L, you are quite simply the bravest, strongest, and most courageous soul I will ever know. You have inspired me and taught me to live my life with courage. I know that I'll never be able to muster up the courage that you showed day in and day out, but I will do my very best in your honor.

I have dreaded this day for over three years. I've gone for long walks, imagining what it would be, what I would say, writing this eulogy in my head and then willing myself to banish the thought. Every day that you woke up in pain, I thought to myself, "How is she going to survive this? How is she going to get through the day?" And every morning, when I came in your room and saw you still there and took your hand in mine, I breathed a sigh of relief.

You deserve so much more from this world than what your body gave you. And if there is one thing I know about you, it's that you will get it, one way or another... you are determined, and you will do all the things in this world you were meant to do. Flesh and blood be damned... they are no match for you.

To all of you here today, I know you all know what I mean. L touched all of you because it was impossible to know her and not be changed by her. Her energy was bigger than anything I've ever known... it took up all the space in the room. It still does. It is so incredibly powerful. I feel it, and I know you all do too. To know L was to know her wit, her sarcasm, her edginess, her depth, her saltiness, her humor, her intellect, her compassion, her tenderness, her insight, her intuition, her dedication, her determination, her curiosity, her charisma, her resilience, her strength, and her love. L didn't do anything half-ass. Be it her fierce protection of her sister, her insatiable quest for knowledge, her dedication to her friends, her ridiculously sharp wit, or her tender moments with the people she loved, there was nothing subtle about L; she was all in, all the time. And to spend even a moment with her was life changing. So many people have reached out to me with stories and memories of L, and I am so deeply honored to know that she touched people in such profound ways.

L, I am amazed by you, I am dazzled by you, I am in awe of you. I don't know how you survived as long as you did in this body of yours that betrayed you in so many ways, that caused you so much pain, but I am so grateful that you did. I'm grateful for every moment that you held on so that I could feel your touch and hear your voice and see you smile. I wish I could keep you here forever, but I know that would be selfish of me to ask you to endure that much pain just so I could have you here.

L, I know you're here right now. I can feel your arms around me. I know you are watching and listening and thanking your lucky stars that you don't have to deal with the crowd. I told you so many times that I would take every ounce of your pain from you so that you could be free. And I know now you are free... so, we'll stay here and hold your pain; you don't have to hold it any more... you just be free. I keep looking up at the sky, and I see your face. I see this huge, smiling L, and it takes up the whole sky... because you're L, so of course you're going to take up the whole sky. I see this smiling face, free from your body, and I know you are soaring! You are riding your bike, and feeling the grass in your toes, and dancing in the rain, and swimming in cool water, and feeling the warmth of the sun and the sand on the beach. I see you; I see you jetting around the world, so light, so free, so pure. I know your soul, your spirit, is doing everything you've wanted to do, everything your body wouldn't let you do. And I'm rejoicing for you... It may not look like it right now, but I promise you, I am.

You often told me one of your biggest fears was dying without having had enough of an impact on this world. L, you have had more of an impact in 15 short years, three of which were largely spent in bed, than anyone I know. With your mind, your curiosity, your relentless pursuit of justice, your heart, your soul, and your computer as your access to the outside world, you have changed people's lives. Most of us are lucky if we are able to impact one, maybe two, maybe three people in our lifetime. L, you have impacted hundreds, if not thousands, and it's only just begun. There is not a person who knew you, there is not a person in this room, who has not been changed by you. That's the power of you. You make us all go deeper, you make us ask the hard questions, you show us what it is like to be brave and fearless, you show us what it is like to be true to our-selves and to live our lives with pride and without fear of judgment. You teach us to look past what we see on the surface and to love people for who they are. You show us how to stand up, or sit down as the case may be, for what is right and to never stop fighting for justice. And in doing all of that, you have changed the world.

So many of you have asked what you can do, how you can help. And all week I've been in a fog, saying, "I don't know." But I do know. For anyone whose life has been touched by L, there is so much you can do. You can savor the taste of Domino's pizza and French fries, you can cherish the feeling of walking on warm sand and rinsing off in cool water. You can be who you are, openly and proudly, and you can fight for what you believe in. You can be a warrior for social justice and equality and humanity. And in doing so, you can help L continue to change this world.

L, I know your heart breaks for me right now, as mine has broken for you for so long. And I'm not gonna lie because you'd see through me in a second if I tried... the grief is unspeakable. But even as I stand here, with a pain that can only be comparable to the pain you felt, I consider myself lucky. Because I get to be your mom. And being your mom and Jaz's mom has been, and will always be, the greatest privilege on this earth. I am honored, I am humbled, I am forever grateful that you chose me as your mom and that I have been loved by you the way I have been loved by you. I am holding you tight in my arms, now and forever, and I will never let you go. I love you more than anything.

Sleep tight, have sweet dreams, call me if you need anything, and know that I love you more every day. I'll see you soon baby girl.

There were hundreds of people in the house for the Shiva by the time we returned from the service. I had promised L's friends, some of whom she had never met in person, that they could spend time in her room, in her space. I found Ashton and got her onto the stairlift so she could join L's other friends upstairs. We got to her room and closed the door behind us, muffling the noise of the crowd as we did. Her friends talked to me about how they met L, how she had become a leader in the Cripple Punk movement, a group that, through Tumblr, came together to support those in the LGBTQ community grappling with disability and chronic illness. One by one, L's friends started to tell me how much she meant to them and how she had, in her own way, quite literally saved each of their lives as they struggled through their own individual illnesses. Eventually, I let them be alone in her space, and I sneaked into Jaz's room and lay next to her for several hours until we had the strength to face the crowds again.

Later, as the last few people were saying their goodbyes, my friend Amy pulled me aside. She was one of the few people who hadn't annoyed me that week. Her intuition was uncanny. She instinctively knew exactly how to show up; she knew exactly what I needed.

"You're going to think I'm crazy, but you are going to start randomly finding dimes. I think it's going to be one of the ways L communicates with you." Her husband looked at her like she was nuts, but she was completely serious. "I'll let you know if I find dimes. I promise." I assured her.

It was close to midnight when the house was finally quiet. Jaz wanted to sleep in her own bed for the first time that week, and I found myself in L's room with my sister. We sat on her bed, too spent to do anything but sit in silence. I glanced at her nightstand, where all her supplements were. I had doled these out every day for years. I had looked at that nightstand every day. There had never been anything on it but supplements. L had not left her room for seven months prior to her passing. And there it was, under a pill cutter: one lone dime.

I started laughing and crying at the same time, my sister sitting next to me utterly baffled. I whipped out my phone and snapped a picture of the dime to send to Amy.

"What is going on?" my sister kept asking.

"I'll tell you in a minute," I laughed, still unable to form a full sentence. When I could finally form words, my sister was dumbfounded. It would be one of the early and many ways that L would continue to talk to us.

I've never been one to journal, but as July 27, 2018, came to an end, I felt compelled to try to express the surreal experience of the day, knowing that if I didn't write it down immediately, I might never be able to fully hold onto the power of the day.

Journal Entry 1
Vanessa Lynn
July 27, 2018

My Sweet Girl,

Today was one of the most extraordinary days... you know it's rare that I write stuff down, and I'll tell you all about it, but I needed to capture it, so that we can always remember.

It actually starts with last night. Agatha came over and Wes arrived for your memorial service. Together they put together a poster for you with pictures of you and so many of the extraordinary friends you made over the past few years. Agatha and Wes, of course, became fast friends, sharing stories and their love for you. Agatha didn't want to leave. She slept in your room just to be close to you.

This morning was your memorial... it doesn't sound like that can even be real, but it was. Amara and her cousin came in also, and they were in the kitchen with Wes when I came downstairs. I got Wes coffee and hazelnut creamer, just like he likes, and we all hugged and cried. Jaz wore your LGBT Docs, and she did it with pride! She's really finding her voice; you would be so proud!

Your memorial was standing room only. There were hundreds of people there—it was literally standing room only. Beside some annoying grand-parent friends, there were so many people there who really, truly, genu-inely cared and just wanted to express their love. Even cooler, there were so many people whose lives you touched and changed. It was amazing. Here's just a few... Mrs. Hechtman, Mr. Leiva, Ms. Sebert, Peter's par-ents, Lev and his family, Madison, Agatha, Wes, Amara, and of course, your biggest fans from my work life, Dick, Tom, David and, wait for it... Donald. I know you would have hated the crowd and all the people, but I swear to you, L, it was amazing to see how many people were so touched by you. The most emotional part was when Ashton showed up. I didn't even know about them (am I getting my pronouns right?). But all

196

of the sudden, this stunning human with blue hair and glasses and a face like yours wheeled into the sanctuary, sobbing. It took my breath away. Here was this beautiful person, who had just learned the night before of your passing, who got on a plane and came to the service and was so absolutely distraught that you were gone. There was something about Ashton, the rawness of their grief, their vulnerability, their beauty, their willingness to be a fish out of water at this service on the North Shore of Chicago to pay respect to you... it just had me floored.

Your service was beautiful. I felt you there the whole time. You were kinda annoyed by all the people, kinda laughing at some of the real doozies, but also taking it all in, and beginning to realize just how much of an impact you've had. I felt your arms around me the whole time. People thought I was crazy to get up and speak, but I have to tell you, it wasn't that hard. Talking about you is easy, and you have given me so much strength.

After the service the house was packed; you would have hated it. But your friends were all there, and we quickly went up to your room. Ashton took the stairlift up... I was so grateful that we had the lift and your wheelchair upstairs so that they could feel comfortable and welcome and know that they could feel at home in our home. Your friends spent time in your room, crying and sharing stories of how much you have saved their lives, over and over. They told me this was just the tip of the iceberg... that there were so many more friends who couldn't make it in but who loved you just the same. Amara told me how you started by asking people who they would want to be on a desert island with and everyone laughed. L, I gotta tell you, something about being with your friends in your room, it just took my breath away. The fact that you were able to build so many deep, meaningful friendships from your bed, the fact that they love you so purely, and that you literally have kept some of them alive... I didn't think it was possible for me to be more proud of you than I already was, but I was blown away. I am awestruck by who you are, what you have done in this world, the quality people you have brought into your world, and the support you have been able to provide others, despite your own pain. All of your friends wanted something of yours so they could keep you with them, and they all loved being in your room. They each took a tee shirt, or a beanie, or a sweatshirt that they could wear, just so they could be close to you. Oh, and Amara took your salt lamp... I told her you had licked it, but she didn't care.

L, your friends are exceptional. And through your life and your passing you were able to bring them together. To see them all together in your room... I just don't even have the words to describe it. I think I am going to try to fly them all in for your sweet 16! Wes didn't want to leave, so we made his flight later. Ashton wants to come back with another one of your friends. Agatha doesn't want to leave your room. It's incredible.

So, Agatha is sleeping in your room again tonight. I gave her our garage code and told her she could stay in your room whenever she would like. She really feels at peace there. I told Wes I'll fly him in any time because he wants to spend more time in your space; I told Ashton to come any time. I love that the house is accessible for them. I could go on and on, but you get my point. Your friends love you so much, they just want to be in your space. And I still am just awestruck that you were able to build these relationships from the confines of your bed, and that you have impacted people the way you have. You are a miracle.

Oh, I forgot to tell you, Lev, Mr. Leiva, Madison, Shall, Peter's parents, they all talked about how you changed their lives. L, you are unbelievable! Mr.

Leiva also said he is a different person because of you.

Sharon came by around 7:00... she had just gotten back from Croatia; I met Rick too. And Melissa came by, and Jessica, the list just goes on. I can't tell you how many people have told me how privileged they are to have known you, and how you have impacted their lives. And some of these people only spent a few moments with you.

Oh, how could I forget... Tom C. stopped by! He was crying and telling me how much he loves you and what a special connection you two had... It was amazing! I want him to be my gay husband.

I could go on and on, but things are starting to get blurry; it's been a long day.

The bottom line is that you need to know how remarkable you are, and how profoundly you have impacted people. I don't have the words to describe it... perhaps the only one who would be able to put it into words is you.

I told all your friends that our home is their home and that I wanted to stay in touch. I am going to keep close to them and try to continue to support them as much as I can.

I've dreaded this day all week, and hard as it was, I walked away even more inspired, even more proud, even more in awe of you... that's not easy to do, but that's what you do to me!!

I can't come close to describing how much I deeply love and respect you. Thank you for being mine.

Oh, and thanks for the dime!!

Goodnight my sweet girl, thanks for making my heart sing.

August 1–7, 2018

Earlier in the spring of 2018, Jaz and I had planned a trip to Grand Cayman.

It was to be a special trip to celebrate her graduation from eighth grade and her entry into high school. L was bedridden when we planned it, but I had booked us at a completely accessible hotel on the remote chance that L would be able to join. L assured me that if she couldn't join, we shouldn't feel bad; after all, it was Grand Cayman, but it wasn't a place she was longing to go to, like Iceland. In the wake of L's death, my initial instinct was to cancel the trip. But after her funeral, it became clear to both me and Jaz that we needed time away; time away from the trauma, time away from all the well-wishers, time to just be. There was a piece of me that felt it was blasphemous somehow to go away, but my friend from Arizona helped me get my head on straight, reminding me of who my daughter was and that she was not one to follow protocol or bow to societal conventions.

"You know she would want you to go and spend time with Jaz, healing," he assured me, "and now, she can go with you."

So, on the morning of August 1, Jaz, Grazer, and I got on a plane and flew to Grand Cayman. We arrived in time for a late lunch, and we munched on salads and fish tacos while they were getting our room ready. Roaming casually by our table were two chickens that would come to join us at every meal. Just before we got up to check on our room, a black bird landed squarely on Jaz's head.

"L!" she exclaimed, "I love you, but come on; you know I'm freaked out by birds!"

It was late in the afternoon by the time we got settled, but the summer sun was still high in the sky, and the beach was beckoning. I had been to the Caribbean several times, but as I stood silently by the shore that afternoon, the water sparkled shades of blue I had never seen before. I took a deep breath and walked closer to the water's edge, squeezing L's hand by squishing my fingers into my palm. "Here we go, sweetheart," I said to her. I came to the intersection of beach and ocean where, if you stand still, you can feel the waves lap at your feet and the warm sand underfoot pull away as the waves are drawn back into the sea. Through my toes I could feel L's toes delighting in the sensation. How long had it been since she had been able to feel the tides gently pulling at her feet? How deeply had she longed to do so? I stayed there for several minutes, still squeezing my fingers to my palm, before Jaz urged me in further.

"The water is so warm, Mom, even you would like it!"

I stepped further in and felt L slip her hand from my grip. "I'm gonna swim now, Momma," I felt her say, "but I won't go far." I could feel her diving headfirst into the water, like a dolphin, making a perfectly formed beeline for the horizon, where the sun was on its path to melt into the sea.

The next day Jaz wanted to go water skiing, so we chartered a boat and were on our way. She was a Rockstar, all the years of camp paying off as she expertly got up on one ski and zigzagged through the water. When she was done, she climbed into the boat, and without us having to ask, the driver took us for a ride, accelerating to full throttle as he headed out to the open sea. Jaz and I sat at the bow of the boat, feeling the exhilaration as our speed increased. We looked at each other and smiled, and without saying a word, we both closed our eyes, tipped our heads back, and spread our arms out wide like Leonardo DiCaprio and Kate Winslet did in *Titanic*. "She's free!" we both cried. It was as if she was inside both of us, impressing upon us her undeniable sense of liberation, her spirit now coursing through our own veins.

We spent the rest of our lazy days there watching the water take on various shades of turquoise and blue while the sun made its way across the sky, rays almost touchable through the occasional cloud. We did not say much, each relishing the solitude and the quiet days to just be with L. When Jaz would go back to the room in the late afternoons to cool off and rest, I would take long walks on the beach, listening to Stevie Nicks and watching hermit crabs burrow into the sand.

At night we'd head down to the pool deck, watch the sunset, and have a casual dinner. On our third or fourth night, we took up our usual post in our favorite waiter's section, and while we were waiting for our food, fireworks erupted over the beach. It took us by surprise at first, but we looked on as the sky lit up with a full fireworks display, a rainbow of sparks sizzling in the sky for 20 minutes, culminating in a grand finale that would rival any Fourth of July display. I was smiling and crying at the same time. Fireworks were one of the few things that L cherished with childhood innocence. It had been four years since she had been able to see fireworks, and as I looked into the Cayman sky I heard L's 15-year-old self, applauding with vigor, and I saw her two-year-old self reaching up to the lights with her chubby hand, as she had 13 years earlier... "More."

The August sun was hot, and on days with no intermittent clouds, it could be scorching. Jaz and I found ourselves, along with most of the hotel guests, in the ocean for hours on a particularly hot day. We had been lucky in snagging a huge foam raft that was anchored to the seafloor, so we could float all afternoon without having to worry about drifting away. Even in the water, the midday summer heat was intense, and as we lay on the raft, we began to feel a small drizzle. We looked up and saw a cloud over our section of ocean, and as the drizzle thickened to a steady rain, all of the hotel guests, including myself and Jaz burst into spontaneous applause, like a flash mob. Collectively, we all noticed that it was only raining over our portion of the beach, and we simultaneously looked up, hundreds of people in unison, thanking the heavens for cooling us off. Nobody left the water. There was no threat of lightning or any danger. It was clear the rain was a gift, and everyone happily splashed around, feeling the freshness of the rain mix with the saltiness of the ocean. Jaz and I leaned back on our raft, eyes closed, bodies rejoicing with the kiss of each rain drop. "Thank you, L," I whispered as we opened our mouths and let the rain fall on our tongues, taking more of L in with each drop.

On August 7th we headed back to Chicago, feeling calmer and more connected to L, steeling ourselves for the reality of what lay ahead. As the plane ascended, I started to nod off, but Jaz tapped me on the shoulder before I fell into a full sleep. "Mom, look..." she pointed out the window. A double rainbow shone bright and proud in the sky.

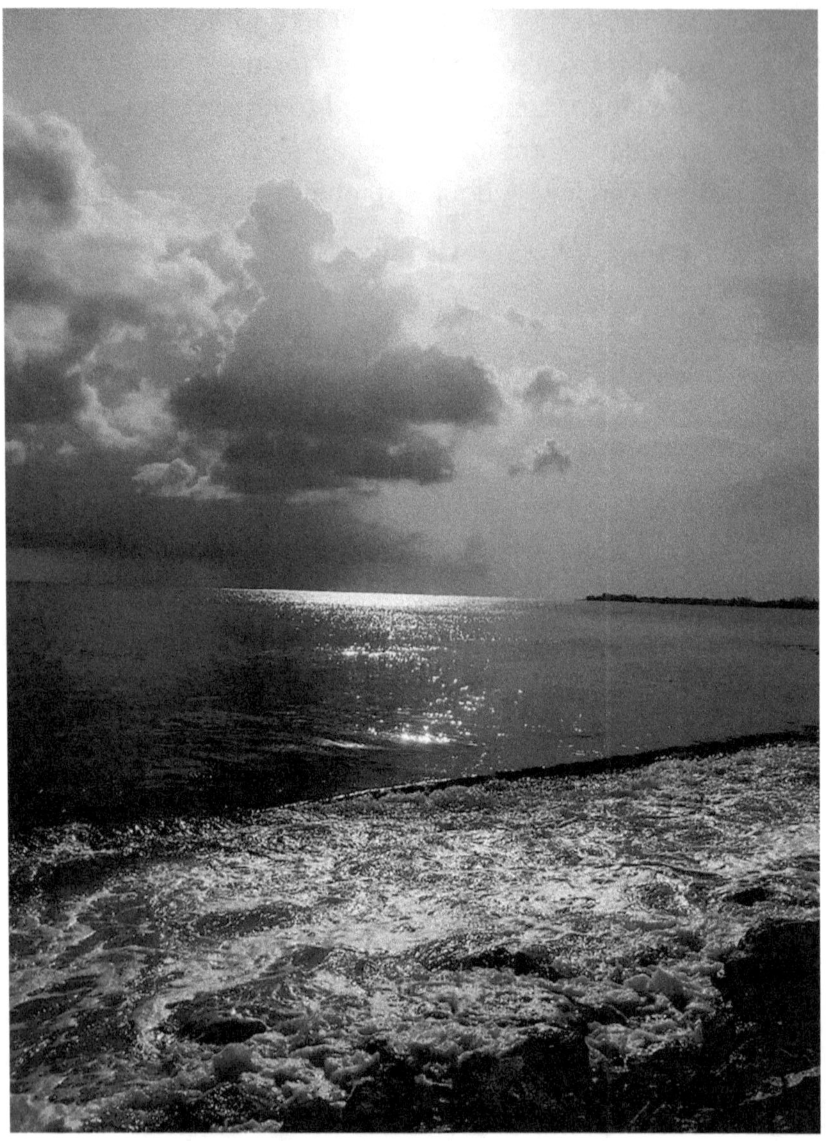

L's energy shining bright in Grand Cayman, August 4, 2018.

August 8, 2018

Coming home was hard, as the vastness of trying to piece together some sort of routine spread out before me. I found myself lying in L's bed, staring up at the star stickers on her ceiling, allowing the grief to wash over me. At some point I sat up and felt compelled to look through her drawers. I'm not sure why. I had opened every drawer, looked at every nook and cranny of her room during "that week," not sure exactly what I was looking for other than anything of hers that I could cling to. But something made me want to look again. I wasn't looking for anything in particular, other than perhaps L. I opened the top drawer of her nightstand. It was completely empty with the exception of one dime. I rubbed it between my finger and thumb, laughing out loud as I cried out, "Thank you, L!"

In the eight months that have passed since her death, I have found myself thanking her out loud every day, often multiple times, for the ways in which she has let me know she is with me. I have collected all the dimes, marking the date, and I keep them in a silver box in my room that Amy gave me. They have always shown up in isolation, never in a pile of change. They have appeared on floormats of cars, as friends have stood up from booths at restaurants, in open fields, under my nose as I've done push-ups at the gym, in old coat pockets, and in the small backpack that L would sling on the back of her wheelchair, floating in her case of anti-nausea medication.

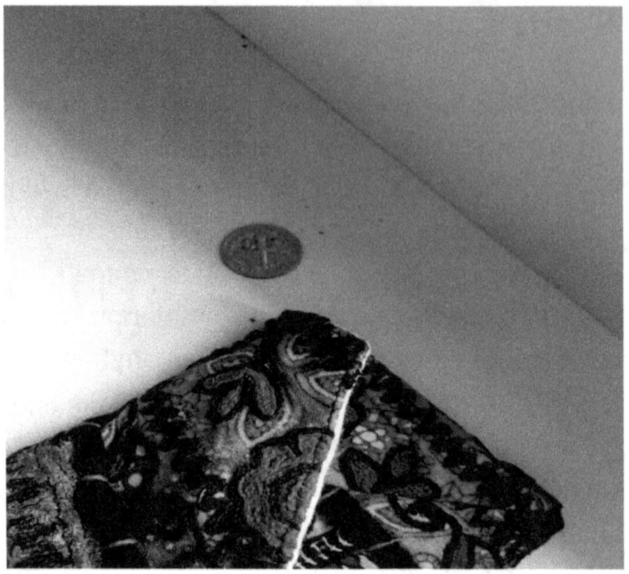

L's nightstand, August 8, 2018.

August 9–September 21, 2018

I had taken a leave of absence from work, and I would be off until October 1. My focus was on making sure Jaz acclimated to high school as smoothly as possible and on reading everything that L wrote—everything she had told me I could only read once she was better but that she made me promise I would help her get published. Jaz had joined cross-country, and practices were early in the morning. I would drive her to school and then head to the beach where I would watch the sunrise. I'd spend the rest of the day alternating between walking for miles and holing up in my office with L's computer until I had read every word she had written. Reading her work was grueling, terrifying, cathartic, and healing all at the same time. I would read until the emotions became too great to contain in my 5'1" frame, then walk for hours, my connection to L strengthening with each step.

L's impact was growing each day and with it the knowledge that her ability to make a difference was not at all hampered by the fact that she was not physically here. At L's funeral, we had asked people who were inclined to make donations to contribute to one of two organizations: One was the Human Rights Campaign (HRC), which fights for equality for the LGBTQ community; the other was the Burning Limb Foundation, a relatively new charity that helps fund treatment for those suffering from CRPS. In the few short weeks since July 22, the Burning Limb Foundation had received so many contributions in L's name that they created the L Grey Memorial Grant, and two young women were already beginning a new treatment regimen. By December of 2018 $90,000 had been raised in L's name.

I knew some people who were close friends with people who were connected to the HRC, and the HRC designated September 7, 2018, as L Grey Day. We flew to Washington, DC, where they gave us a private tour of their office and allowed us into their media room where we each wrote L a message on the wall in permanent marker, her name and her story becoming an indelible part of their fabric. They flew a flag in her honor and took us up to the roof just so we could touch it. The same yellow equal sign against a blue background that decorated her computer case now waved proudly in the DC summer heat, fueled, unequivocally, by L's spirit.

As August gently turned to September, I found myself increasingly conflicted. I felt as if every one of my senses was heightened, like I was seeing and experiencing the world in technicolor. Everything was brighter. I saw colors I had never seen before. I saw sunrays stream through the clouds on even the gloomiest of days, almost begging me to touch them. Rainbows popped up everywhere—in the sky, in my kitchen, and in my dining room. I would get in the car and "Dream On," "Don't Stop Believin'," "Another One Bites the Dust," and dozens of Fleetwood Mac songs would come on the radio with surprising frequency. Food started to taste better. Jaz noticed it too. We were sitting on the couch, eating some freshly made gluten-free brownies, and neither of us could get over how good they were.

"Jazzy, I know this may sound strange, but does food taste better to you?" I asked.

"YES! I thought it was just me, but I swear, everything tastes different. It's like everything I eat is the best thing I've ever tasted."

I could literally feel L in me, giving me a glimpse of the brightness and beauty of the world she was in and reminding me, through a constant gentle buzzing in my legs, of the world she had left. The strength of her energy is what buoyed me through those days and is what carried me in the months that would follow.

Coupled with the warmth of feeling her spirit was the melancholy sense of fall in the air. The nights became crisp, and the leaves were turning brown (actually, the leaves on the big cottonwood tree in our front yard turned brown the day L died). Fall was L's favorite season. She had desperately wanted to be outside, to feel leaves underfoot and inhale the crispness of the air mingled with an occasional campfire smell. There was a part of me that was so joyful at the thought of L being able to experience fall in her own way, free from her pain. And there was a part of me that was distraught that she could not be physically here to experience it. "She needs to be here," I would think to myself. "She needs to be here for this. How can she not be here?" My thoughts would then turn to what the reality would be had she been here, lying flat in bed gasping for breath, body on fire, feet bleeding, heart beating out of her chest, watching the leaves fall outside her window. "How could she possibly bear to watch another season pass from the confines of her bed and the confines of her body?" I would think. It was an impossible, vicious loop in my head. I could not bear her not being here to experience the change of seasons. My body ached for her. And I could not bear the thought of her being here and suffering.

Surrounding all of this was the realization that time was passing—it would not stay that warm July day forever; we were moving from the season of her death to the season of... I didn't know what. I just knew that the coming of fall loomed ominous in my mind and body. I could feel it, and I cautioned my family and close friends that the coming weeks would likely be particularly difficult for me. "I'm going to need a lot of solitude; don't take it personally" I warned them. I felt more off kilter with each passing day of September, the autumnal equinox barreling toward me like a tornado.

September 22, 2018

It was homecoming at the high school, and Jaz and her friends made a lastminute decision to go. Jaz was radiant, and we gathered at the house of one of her friends to take pictures. I was filled with so much pride for Jaz. She had been through the unthinkable, yet she always maintained an ability to find joy in the moment and to love with her whole heart. When I had snapped every picture from every possible angle, I kissed her goodbye and got in my car to go home.

About a block into the drive, I found myself turning left, even though I should have headed right to get to my house. I was headed to the beach. I hadn't planned it, but it was undoubtedly where I was going. As I pulled into the parking lot, I glanced out the driver's side window and saw the moon beginning to rise over Lake Michigan. I flung my car door open and, drawn by a force as strong as gravity, started running toward the shoreline as if my whole existence depended it, whispering, "Oh my God, L," under my breath. To anyone watching me, I was simply running to the shore, eager to watch a beautiful moonrise, but in my soul, I was running toward L. I was breathless when I got to the water's edge, overcome by what I saw.

The sky to the east was a palette of pastels, the purple of the horizon giving way to pink, orange, yellow, and pale blue. The full moon sat in the center, glowing pure white. Behind me, to the west, the sky glowed a deep ruby as the sun was setting. I took out my phone, knowing the camera could not possibly convey the beauty or passion of the moment, but needing to document it nonetheless. It was only when I took out my phone to snap photos that I noticed the day and time. September 22, 6:45 pm. It was the autumnal equinox. I had somehow found myself at the beach at the exact moment that summer turned to fall, the full moon rising over the water as the sun set behind the trees. L's presence was so palpable it took my breath away. She was everywhere, and my whole body pulsed with the burst of her energy. Unable to speak or move, I stood watching the moon continue to climb, taking in every ounce of L that I could. It was indescribable. It was transcendent. The angst that had been growing all month immediately evaporated, replaced with an electricity that coursed through me and a deep, deep knowing that L was not just out of pain. She was thriving.

Moonrise over Lake Michigan, September 22, 2018.

September 26, 2018

In the two months since L had died, five different people in my life, none of whom knew each other, called me to tell me I needed to meet with Lisa Nitzkin. I had never heard her name before, but she was touted as a gifted medium, and those who knew L and me felt it was imperative that I talk with her. I was open to the idea, but her website said she was booked for months and offered no available appointments. Unbeknownst to me, these women, and some of their friends whom I didn't even know, had been trying behind the scenes to get me in. But Lisa had a strict rule that she would not see anyone until at least six months had gone by since someone had passed. Her boundaries were firm. Finally, at Amy's emphatic insistence, in conjunction with my cousin's sister-in-law's begging, Lisa agreed to see me on October first. No one had told her anything about me other than the fact that she needed to bend her rules. In retrospect, we would all agree that the person who actually made sure Lisa and I met was L. She was going to pull out all the stops, and she was not going to back down until Lisa surrendered.

On September 26th I was walking along the beach with Amy.

"I know you've got an appointment with Lisa coming up," she said. "In the meantime, she's teaching a class on meditation, mindfulness, and intuition. I've been wanting to take the class for years, but the timing never seemed right until now. In any case, it starts tomorrow and meets every Thursday for five weeks. You should come. I think it's really important you meet her as soon as possible. I just have this feeling that she's someone you need to know."

"I'd love to, but I'm going back to work soon. I don't know if I could commit to a five-week class. You know my schedule is going to get busy really fast." "Why don't you come to just the first class tomorrow and see what you think? I know it sounds nuts, but something tells me you need to meet her *now*."

I trusted Amy. Completely. The day after L passed, she showed up at the bottom of my stairs, and after a long, tearful hug, she sprang to action, planning for the Shiva and delivering smoothies to Jaz, instinctively knowing what to do. She was in tune with me in a way very few people were. "Okay," I agreed. "I'll be there."

September 27, 2018

The drive to Lisa's house took four minutes, just enough time for "Don't Stop Believin'" to randomly come on the radio, the last few chords fading behind the DJs voice as I pulled into her driveway. I walked in and was immediately at ease in the tranquility of her living room. The silver velvet couches, sheer white drapery, and crystal mirrors created a mini oasis in suburban Chicago. We caught each other's eye and instantly embraced, though I had not yet even told her my name. "I'm so glad you're here," she said.

It was a small group of about six or seven women, and we quickly made ourselves at home in her living room. Lisa introduced herself and the purpose of the class, her hope being that it would help each of us be more in touch with our own intuition. She then talked about how she came to understand her own gifts as a medium. Her story began with her mother's cancer diagnosis and ultimate passing when Lisa was seven years old. Her mother, Lisa told us, would always show up in rainbows. Every holiday, every major life event, no matter the weather, a rainbow would appear. I tucked this in my mind as Lisa continued to talk about her journey into mediumship and the years she spent honing her craft. The other women in the class then introduced themselves, talking openly about their own experiences and what they hoped to learn. I happened to be last, and when it was my turn, I was careful not to say much. I had an upcoming private session with Lisa, and I didn't want to reveal anything that might bias that. I kept things short and simple.

"I lost my daughter over the summer," was all I said. I then shifted my attention to Amy, who was sitting next to me. I began explaining what a tremendous friend Amy had been to me when Lisa suddenly stood up from her chair, "I'm so, so sorry to interrupt you. I hate to be rude, but your daughter is yelling so loudly in my ear right now."

Lisa began walking toward me, the whole room in a breathless hush.

"She is saying, 'Give my mom the necklace, give my mom the necklace, let her know I'm okay.'" She continued moving toward me, her hands behind her head as she removed a small gold and crystal rainbow necklace from her neck.

"I don't know what this means, but she is insisting I give this to you," she said as she reached behind my head to fasten the gold rainbow around my neck. I stood shaking, eyes closed, as she secured the clasp, placing the necklace against my chest the same way the nurses had placed L on my chest the night she was born. All of the air had left the room, and, for a moment, time stood completely still. Lisa and I hugged deeply as the tears streamed down my face. "I promised myself I wouldn't cry," I whispered.

The other women in Lisa's living room sat in complete stillness, unable to move or take a full breath. Their jaws were slack, and their cheeks were stained with their own tears. None of us, including Lisa, was sure what to do next.

"What just happened?" It was Amy who broke the silence.

"I'm not sure," Lisa said. "I've never had a message that clear or strong, and I've never been compelled to give away a personal belonging. Your daughter's energy is incredible! She was not going to shut up until I gave you that necklace. Do rainbows mean something to you, or to her?" "When she died, she told me she would be in every rainbow..." For the second time that morning, all of the air left the room.

Three hours later, when class ended, Lisa and I waited for the others to leave so we could have a private moment.

"I don't know what to say. I don't know how to thank you. I'm speechless," I kept repeating.

"Your daughter is amazing, and she has a lot to say. And I have a feeling I have a lot to learn from her. She is going to help me in my work. You're coming back Monday morning. We have a lot to talk about."

"I kinda feel like all I want to do is sit on your couch and talk to L."

I got in my car, still dizzy from the whole experience; I tried to ground myself for the short drive home. As I pulled out of her driveway, "Dream On" came on the radio. "Thank you, L!" I shouted at the top of my lungs. "Thank you!" Steven Tyler's voice carried me the rest of the way, the force of L as strong as it had been the day she was born.

Sing with me,
Sing for the year,
Sing for the laughter, and sing for the tear,
Sing with me if it's just for today, maybe tomorrow the good lord will
take you away...

September 29, 2018

"Did L like Tom Petty?" my sister asked.

"I'm not sure. I love him. I don't know if she was a huge fan, but I hope she's hanging out with him now. He seems like a cool guy."

"I love him too. Can't you picture them rocking out together?"

I smiled. "I can totally see them writing lyrics together and jamming." "Maybe he's teaching her how to play guitar." "I love that image," I said. "Me too."

September 30, 2018

"Mommy," Jaz was tentative, but she clearly had something she wanted to ask me. "I'm ready to go back to Soul Cycle. Can we go?"

"Of course, we can, sweetheart."

"Are you sure? Will you be okay?" She had grown quite protective of me.

"I'll be fine, lovey. I think it will be good to be back."

We walked into the same Sunday morning class we had been in over two months earlier. Though our world was totally different, the studio looked the same, which somehow surprised me, as if it too should have changed alongside us. We clipped into our bikes as Dylan entered the dark room.

"We're going to do something a little different today." He was doing his Sunday morning motivational speech. "We're going to change it up from our typical music. But just go with me. Trust me. Trust the music. Just listen and ride to the beat. This is a live recording, so there's some talking at the beginning, but just take it all in. You'll feel it when the music starts." Tom Petty's voice then filled the room as he introduced a live version of "The Waiting (is the hardest part)," the crowd for whom he was playing going wild as he let loose on his guitar. Inside the studio, we collectively started pedaling to the rhythm as I laughed out loud and smiled up at L. Dylan kept the energy going throughout class, ending his playlist with a rocked-out version of "Amazing Grace." "This is for all the mothers and daughters and sisters," he said, blowing out the candles so that we ended our ride in peaceful darkness.

I felt compelled to introduce myself to him after class. Jaz and I had taken several classes with him that past spring, but he didn't know us or anything about us, and I felt like he needed to know about the gift he had given. I approached him as the crowds thinned. "I'm Vanessa,"

I held out my hand. "You wouldn't know this, but you just created an amazing space for me and my daughter Jaz." He smiled. "I promise this isn't a sob story, but I need to tell you this…" I proceeded to give him an abbreviated version of L's story, telling him how we had been in his class the day of her passing, how this was our first day back, how my sister and I had talked about her hanging out with Tom Petty the day before, and how, without even knowing it, he had made our return to class not only safe, but magical and alive with L's spirit. His eyes filled with tears. "Two years ago, I was a heroin addict. I wasn't going to make it. And somehow, I found my way. All I want to do is come into this studio and impact someone's life in a positive way. Your telling me L's story is going to keep me going for a long, long time."

Since hearing "The Waiting" in class that day, there is not a single day that has gone by that my sister or I (often both of us) have not heard a Tom Petty song randomly come on the radio. Not one day. As I write this it has been six months since that September day. And each day my sister and I have texted each other photos of our dashboards, displaying whatever Tom Petty song happened to come on. Some days there were a half-dozen texts. We've heard familiar songs like "Free Fallin," "Runnin' Down a Dream," "The Waiting," "Don't Come around Here No More," "You Don't Know How It Feels," "You Wreck Me," and "Won't Back Down." We've heard songs we never knew before, like "Wildflowers," "Keep a Little Soul," "Dark Side of the Sun," "Free Girl Now," "Angel Dreams," "Have Love, Will Travel," "Time to Move On," and "You and I Will Meet Again." We've looked up the lyrics and have been more amazed with each new discovery; every song carrying a deep message, as if the lyrics, most of which had been written decades before L was born, were somehow written for her.

October 1, 2018

"Another One Bites the Dust" was playing on the radio as I drove back to Lisa's house. I arrived at 10:00 that morning, finding her living room just as soothing as it had been four days prior. We sat together on her couch, and I turned on the voice recorder of my phone.

Lisa's words came out in an almost frenetic pace. "I have L standing here. She's telling me how much she loves you. She's saying she had a hard time breathing prior to her passing. She keeps saying she had a hard time breathing but that's gone. She's talking about dying around her sister's birthday. She's so sorry about this, but she is saying she doesn't feel trapped in her body anymore, and she's thanking me desperately for saying this to you. She's saying her body was... I don't understand this, except to say that her body was... she's showing me like almost frozen. I don't really know what this means, except to say that she doesn't feel trapped in her body anymore, and it's a huge message I'm supposed to tell you. Do you understand this message?"

The session went on like this for three hours, specific details of L's childhood, the progression of her illness, and her ultimate decision to end her pain being revealed as we talked. "You guys could communicate without even having to speak, she's showing me, like you could read each other's minds. Did you have a premonition that she was going to take her life?" she asked. "She's showing me that you had a knowing, not consciously, but that your premonition is what gave her the peace to know that it was going to be okay... and she's thanking you." Lisa paused and breathed deeply as I sat quietly crying. "There is a big *thank you*. It makes me want to cry...too." "I wish I could have held her," I whispered.

"You did. Energetically you did. You don't even know it, but she's telling me you did. She felt you."

Lisa went on and talked to me about L's relationships with me, her sister, her aunt, and her grandparents with eerie specificity. "She wants her sister to know how sorry she is for everything her sister has had to go through, and what a good job she is doing handling things. She's being such a big sister and messing with her, like hiding her things and stuff, but she's having fun with it!"

She talked about her incomparable intellect, used expressions that were uniquely L, recited lines from poems L had written, displayed L's physical mannerisms, and referenced L's final request of where she wanted her ashes spread (Sanibel Island) from the note she left me on July 22. But it was bigger than that. Bigger than anything I can express in words. L's personality, her humor, her wit, her sass, all of it was right there, fully intact. It was in the room with us, and the only way I could describe it is to say it was like spending three hours having brunch with L. Lisa and I would laugh out loud at her jokes and be floored by her insight, prompting Lisa to ask within the first few minutes of our session, "Was she feisty? Cuz she is challenging me!"

The time I spent on Lisa's couch that morning was miraculous, and I feel, even as I am writing this, that I am not coming close to doing it justice. I don't think I possibly could. It confirmed for me, in unmistakable, perfect detail what I knew to be true: that L was happy and joyful, that her work had only just begun, that her impact would continue to grow stronger each day, that she wasn't really gone, that my relationship with her was not a thing of the past but was current and continuing to evolve, and that she and I would be together forever.

October 6, 2018

Wes had texted me a few weeks prior to let me know that Fleetwood Mac was going to be performing in Chicago. He knew how much L and I loved Stevie Nicks, and he thought I might want to go. I immediately bought tickets for myself and my sister, and on that Saturday night we headed out to the United Center, knowing it is where L wanted us to be. The lights dimmed, and the crowds began to cheer as the evocative guitar opening of "The Chain" filled the stadium... "Ladies and gentlemen," the announcer's voice boomed, "Fleetwood Mac!" Within minutes, thousands of people were singing in unison... *We will never break the chain.*

The concert was spectacular. I could feel L there with us. The audience would not leave without an encore, and after a quick break at the end of the last set, Stevie and the band returned to the stage. They began to play a very familiar tune, but it was not their own. It was Tom Petty. The crowd went crazy as they recognized the distinctive first notes of "Free Fallin'." My sister and I locked eyes as Stevie belted out the homage to her dear friend, clearly being carried by Tom's energy as much as we were being carried by L's; the poignancy of Tom's lyrics, sung with the passion of Stevie's voice, creating a tidal wave of emotion.

I'm gonna write her name in the sky,
I'm gonna free fall out into nothing,
I'm gonna leave this world for a while...

October 12, 2018

It was two weeks before my birthday. I was walking on a warm but overcast fall morning, watching the sun peek out from behind the clouds, when I felt the clasp on the rainbow necklace that Lisa had given me break. To my surprise, I didn't panic or take it as an omen. I simply caught the necklace in the collar of my sweatshirt and put in my pocket, making a mental note to bring it into a jewelry store to get it fixed. Later that afternoon, as I was pulling out from the drive-thru at the bank near my house, I remembered that there was a jewelry store in the strip mall adjacent to the bank. I wasn't sure if it was still there, but as I looked around the corner, I saw the sign for it and figured it was as good a place as any to get the clasp fixed. Although the store was just blocks from my house, I had never been there; it's not often that I buy myself jewelry. I walked in and asked if they could fix the clasp and began window-shopping, looking at the display of diamonds while they worked on it. Out of the corner of my eye, I saw a necklace in the display case with a name written in black diamonds. Something made me do a double take, and I approached the case to see it up close. Glistening in front of me, in beautiful black diamonds, I could clearly read L's full given name in cursive. I summoned the store owner over and asked to take a closer look.

"Did you make this for someone?" I asked.

"No," she said. "I had never done a name before and I wanted to try one. This name just came to me over the summer. At first, I did it in white diamonds, but that didn't feel right. Then I tried the black diamonds, and that did the trick."

I quickly told her about L, and by the time I was done, she had come out from behind the display case and had her arms tenderly wrapped around me. "I think I need that necklace. L just gave me my birthday present." I left the store that afternoon with L's name sparkling on my chest, resting just above the fixed and freshly polished gold rainbow.

October 21, 2018

Jaz was in San Antonio to celebrate her cousin's bat mitzvah, and I took the weekend to visit my friend Donna and her family in Florida. Donna and I could go months without talking and pick up exactly where we left off when we reconnected. She understood me. She understood L. And she could always, always make me laugh. It was good to be in her space. But, flying home, I felt myself overwhelmed with how much I missed L's physical presence. I sat on the plane, looking at pictures of her in the hospital, reminding myself of how much she suffered, as if that could somehow make her absence more tolerable. At one point I looked up from my phone to clear my head of pictures of

IVs and lesions and scars. I looked out the window and saw the largest rainbow I had ever seen. It wasn't actually a rainbow *in* the sky, the rainbow *was* the sky. The sun was setting in such a way that the deep garnet red of the horizon released itself to a vibrant orange, followed by yellow and green. As my gaze traveled further up, the green melted into a pale blue and then lavender, culminating in a deep, royal indigo. Of course, I took a picture, determined to capture every image of L I possibly could.

I sat back in my seat, looking at the picture I had just taken, trying to wrap my head around the message I knew L was sending me. I accidentally learned that if you are looking at a picture on an iPhone and you scroll down, the phone will automatically show images of "related" photos—photos that some algorithm determines to be similar to the one you are looking at. I hadn't known this (I'm technically remedial), but my thumb must have accidentally scrolled down because I was suddenly looking at a photo "related' to the rainbow sky. It was a picture of L at age nine, perfectly healthy, smiling wide, and giving two thumbs up to the camera. I couldn't believe what I was seeing. There was nothing at all on the surface of these two images that was "related" in any way. Except, of course, that they were both pictures of L. She was determined to let me know that she was not that sick child unconscious in a hospital bed that I had been crying over. She was the vibrant girl with two thumbs up, illuminating the entire sky.

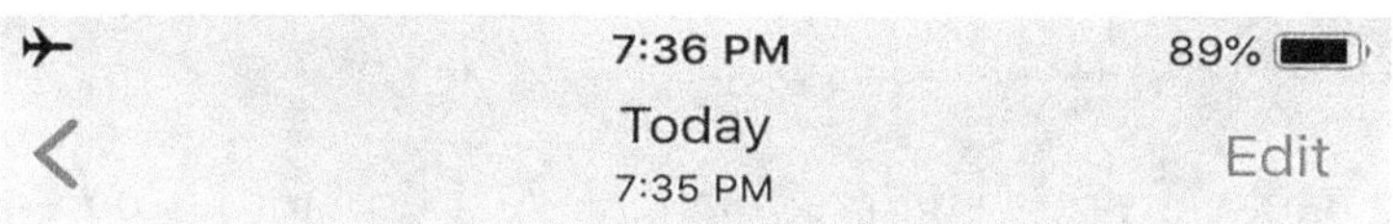

Effects

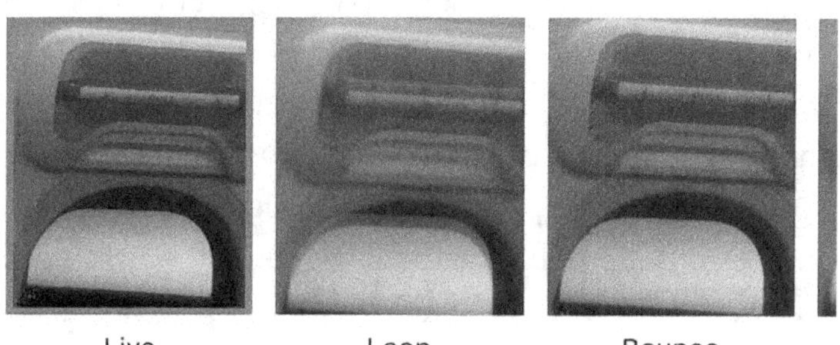

Related

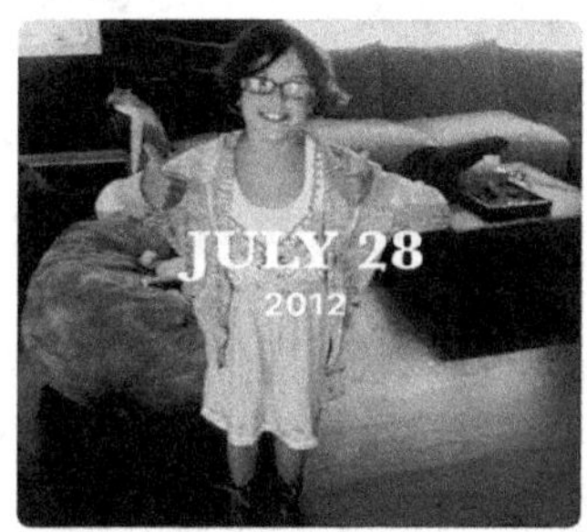

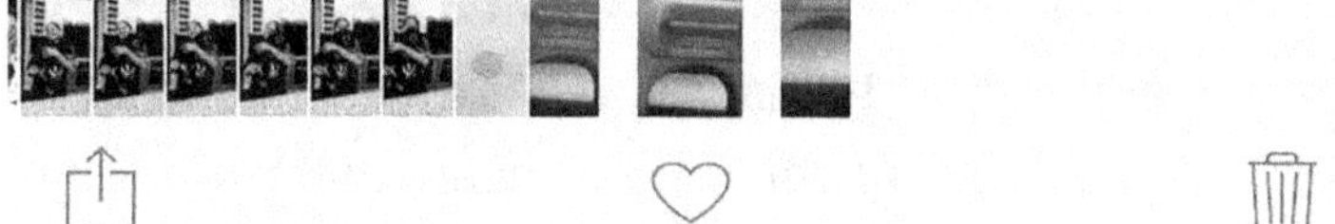

October 30, 2018

My dad was not a spiritual man. He lost both of his parents at a young age and grew up believing that the end is the end, that there is nothing beyond the flesh. Earlier in October, before he was heading off to Asia for three weeks, he stumbled upon an article in the *Chicago Tribune* about an up-and-coming local author. Her name was Eve L. Ewing, and the book was called *Ghosts in the Schoolyard*. There was a small photo of the author, and my dad thought that she looked like L. So, not having any idea what the book was about, he decided he would download it on his kindle and read it on the long flight over the Pacific. He returned from Asia on October 30th a changed man in more ways than one. The book, as it turned out, was about the history of segregation and institutional racism in the city of Chicago and explained the invisible factors that perpetuated the cycle of poverty and poor education. It outlined, with perfect clarity, what L had been trying to get my dad to understand for years during their friendly but heated debates.

"I get it," he admitted. "I get what L has been trying to tell me. I see it now. And I know it was no coincidence that I found this book. I know she guided me to it." It was a profound realization, not just because he began to see institutional racism through different eyes, but because he began to think differently about life and death and spirituality. It was becoming clear that the lessons L was here to teach and the role she was here to play in our lives were not dependent on her physical body. She was determined to teach us what we needed to learn and to do the work her soul was meant to do. The fact that she was not physically here did not seem to faze or deter her in the least. I could almost hear her voice saying, "Mom, I just don't have a body. Like that's gonna stop me from doing what I want to do?!? Seriously, it's no big deal. Everyone needs to chill out. I'm still right here." And so, with L's not so gentle guidance, I watched my stubborn 75-year-old father's belief system shift before my eyes. Gone was the man who believed that dead and buried meant gone for good. He was replaced with someone open to the intangible and un-seeable; someone who, in the months to come, would develop a deep sense of spirituality. "Only L," I said to my sister. "There is no other force on earth that would be strong enough to change Dad's mind about anything!" We laughed because it was just so very true.

November 10, 2018

I had been planning L's sweet 16 for several weeks. After all, a promise is a promise, and we shook on it. The owner of DMK is a friend of mine from high school, and when I called to ask if he might be able to hold a table for us, he responded with his signature generosity. "Just let me know how many people will be coming. We'll take care of everything else," he assured me. So, on Saturday night, November 10, two days prior to L's official 16th birthday, a table for 15 people was set at DMK. Although L had originally joked about having four people, there were too many people who wanted to come and honor her to cap it at that. We had a motley crew of family, friends, teenagers, and adults, many of whom had traveled to be there for L. David, the restaurant owner, had our table decorated with rainbow ribbons, glitter, and personalized menus that read "In honor of L Grey's Sweet 16." We spent the evening stuffing ourselves with burgers, cheddar fries, and milk shakes, just as L had requested. I hope she had fun. I think she did.

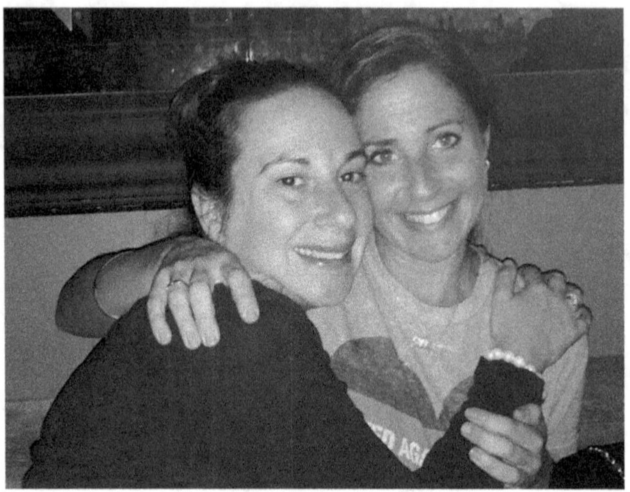

Me and "D" at L's Sweet 16.

November 12, 2018 (L's 16th birthday)

I wasn't sure how I would feel, but I knew that one way or another L would help me through the day. I woke up and began making my way to the kitchen to start the day, passing through my dining room to do so. The sun was streaming through the window, dancing off the crystal chandelier. It cast no fewer than a dozen rainbows in the dining room that morning. They appeared on the walls, on the painting that hung above the breakfront, on the ceiling, and on the floor. One formed in the shape of the letter "L." I reached out my hand to touch it, knowing that we would make it through the day okay.

It was early, and Jaz was still in bed, so I laced up my shoes and headed out for a run. With my playlist of "L" songs on shuffle, I headed out into the cool morning air with a clear head, open and waiting for what L would tell me. I began to run and found that my legs, which usually started burning immediately, felt weightless under me. I pushed my pace, gaining speed with each step, but I was still weightless, barely able to feel the ground beneath me. My breath did not come quick and short, the way it usually did when I was running; I breathed in full, deep, slow breaths with each step, never once feeling winded. I ran, weightless, for six miles that morning. In the background, music was streaming through my headphones. In the foreground, L was telling me, "Momma, I took my life *back*! I'm home!"

Jaz and I spent the rest of the day together. We each took a small glass jar and filled it with a note for L. Jaz also put some M&Ms and L's favorite rainbow lollipops that she had ordered in bulk from China (how had I not noticed that before?!?) in her jar. "I know she can't really eat them, but they're her favorite," Jaz proclaimed with pride. We then went to the beach and set our jars afloat on the water as we wished L a happy birthday.

From there we headed downtown; we were on a mission. Three hours later, when we returned home, I had a tattoo of a flame on my left ankle and the words *True Love Always Liberates the Beloved* forever inscribed on my forearm.

Later that night, when Jaz was in bed, I found myself in L's room with a large trash bag. I had not had the will to remove anything from her room in the months since her passing, and it still looked more like a hospital room than a teenage girl's bedroom. I knew that at some point my body would let me know when it was ready to remove saline bags, catheters, heparin flushes, and IV poles, and that to try to force it before I was ready would be futile. In the last few hours of her birthday, my body felt ready. It was not a conscious thought. It was nothing I'd planned. I just found myself in there throwing away medical supplies that could not be used by anyone else and making a separate pile of things that could be donated. I kept everything else intact— her bed, the clothes in her closet, the books on her shelf, the candles on her nightstand, the soap and shampoo and makeup in her bathroom. It was still L's room, and her stuff belonged there, but her sickness did not.

It was nearing midnight when I opened the last of the drawers in her bathroom vanity to see if there was anything I should throw away. Behind some unraveled gauze bandaging I saw a yellow sticky note. I moved the gauze aside and noticed that resting on top of it was a ring of white gold with a small yellow-gold heart in the center. The ring had been mine in high school. I hadn't seen it or thought about it in 30 years, but it had been sitting somewhere at the bottom of a small velvet box in the chest in my room where I keep my jewelry. And L must have found it. On the sticky note L had written, "I knew you'd find it. Just to be clear, in case you were wondering, I'm right here. Always have been, always will be. Love you." I placed the ring on my finger, stacked on top of my grandmother's wedding ring and the birthstone ring L had given me for Mother's Day.

L's signature, November 12, 2018, her Sweet 16.

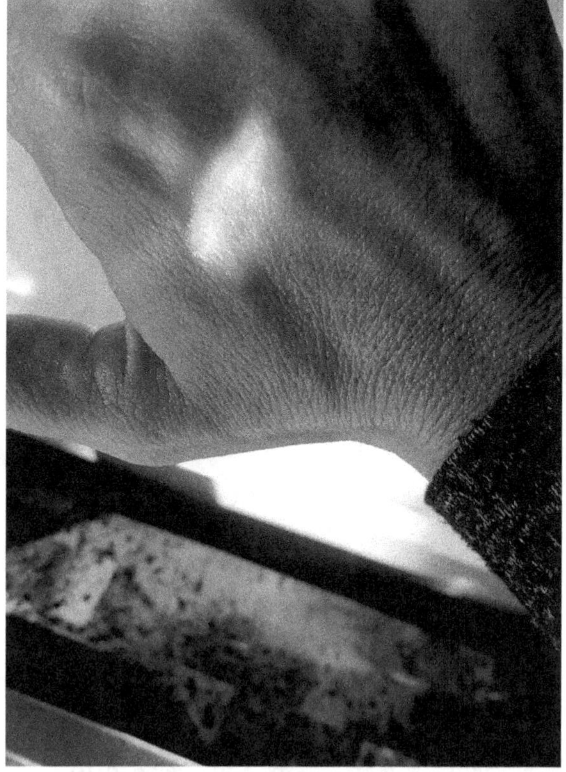

L holding my hand, November 12, 2018.

November 17, 2018

It was the first snow of the season, and I woke up to find a text of a photo from my sister, which, in and of itself, was not unusual. We had been texting photos of songs on the radio, twigs shaped like perfect L's, blackbirds in flight, and rainbows materializing in some ridiculously mundane places multiple times a day. But this text was different. The night before we had been reading L's poem *10,000*, the one that ends with the line, *We can bloom in the snow*. The text I woke up to was taken while my sister was out walking her dog that morning. Two perfect purple petunias were standing up tall in a lawn completely blanketed in snow.

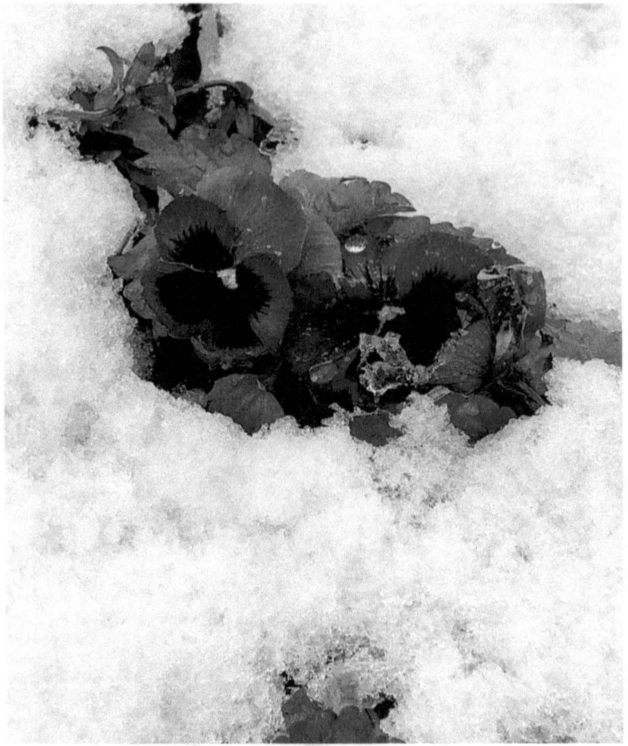

Sent to me by "D," November 17, 2018.

November 20, 2018

I was standing in the foyer of an office building, preparing to facilitate a meeting, and I ran into a client whom I had not seen since I had returned to work. She was more than a client, actually; I'd consider her a friend. She was clearly relieved to see me standing upright and eager to hear how I was doing. It was a cold November day, and the two of us stood talking in the lobby with our coats still zipped tight, hands buried in our pockets to try to get feeling back in our fingers. As I tried to quickly summarize the journey I had been on in the four months since L's passing, I found myself telling her the story of the lone dime that appeared on her nightstand the evening of her memorial service and the subsequent dimes that would follow. Her eyes misted over.

She reached her hand out of her coat pocket and breathed deeply, "I've been fidgeting with this since we started talking," she gave me a crooked smile. "I think this must be for you," she said, as she placed a single dime in my hand.

December 29, 2018

Jaz, Grazer, and I were in Sanibel Island along with my sister, my dad, and my stepmother, as we had been for so many years. It was, of course, a bittersweet time filled with memories of L, signs of her presence, and our collective longing to just be able to hold her. I couldn't help but think back to the last time we had all been there the year before. It had been L's last trip, just before the surgery that left her confined to her bed. As a child, she had always felt at peace in Sanibel, but her last trip was mostly consumed with pain and fear. I knew she was once more at peace, and I had no doubt she had asked for her ashes to be spread in the ocean there so she could hold onto that childhood happiness for eternity.

Jaz was not ready to officially spread L's ashes. She needed her winter break to be a true break, an escape from everything heavy, a time for her to just breathe. I understood that. And yet, I felt compelled to at least bring some of L's remains with me to release into the ocean while we waited for the right time to do something more ceremonial. I brought a small portion of her ashes with me, thinking I would know if and when the time was right to privately scatter them.

I woke up on December 29th and knew that was the day. It marked the one-year anniversary of the surgery, and it seemed fitting that, one year from the day of her ultimate confinement, she be set free. I decided I would spread her ashes at sunset. The morning was particularly foggy; foggier, in fact, than I had ever seen it. I set off on my morning walk, knowing I needed to gear up for what the evening would hold. The fog on the beach was so thick I could barely see in front of me, the ocean and the sand becoming one. My skin and hair were wet from the fog, the dampness cleansing my body and mind. I looked out over the ocean on my right, and then turned to try to make out the trees to my left. The fog had just begun to lift, and glimmers of sun were coming through. Surrounding the trees in a perfect arc was a distinct "white rainbow" of fog. I had never (and have not since) seen anything like it. I stood still, mesmerized by what I was seeing. I wanted to keep walking, but I was enchanted by the sight, and, thinking it would vanish at any moment, I did not want to miss one second of it. I felt L slip her fingers between mine. "Come on, Mom, I'll walk with you," she said. I pressed my fingers into my palms as I had in Grand Cayman to secure her grip in mine and slowly began walking. I took tentative steps, keeping my eyes on the white rainbow, thinking surely it was going to disappear. But it didn't. It grew crisper, more distinct with each step. I could see where the fog met the ground on both sides of the arc, and as I moved along the beach, so too did the arc and its endpoints. I decided I would walk for as long as the rainbow was there, much like I had decided to walk for as long as L slept in her Baby Björn on that fall day 15 years before. I walked for two-and-a-half hours that morning, my fingers intertwined with L's, the white rainbow staying by my side every step of the way.

In the afternoon Jaz and I took a break from the sun and went inside to watch some TV.

"Do you mind if we watch SpongeBob?" she asked.

"I love SpongeBob."

Nickelodeon played some of our classic favorites. "Squid's Day Off," "Band Geeks," and "The Fry Cook Games."

That evening I invited my sister down to the beach with me, and we sat quietly together as the sun sank lower in the sky. When it began to duck behind the horizon, I took the small portion of L's ashes in my hands, held her to my lips, and then released her into the waves. I could hear her voice. "Thank you, Momma," she said.

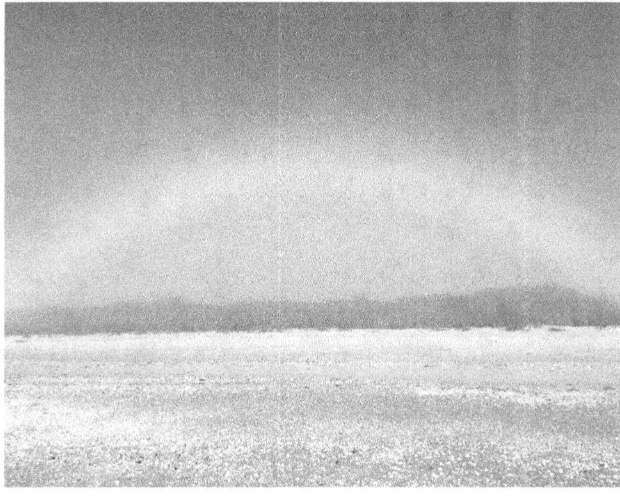

Sanibel Island, Dec 29, 2018.

January 2019–February 2019

Winter brought a surprising calm. Though the days were short, and it was bitter cold, L found ways every day to let me know she was with me. I had come to quickly recognize her signs, and while they were familiar, they took my breath away every time. Never one to rest on her laurels, L also peppered her usual ways of letting me know she was here with novel ways, each one seeming more unbelievable than the last. Each one filling me with more amazement and gratitude.

January 19, 2019

I dreamt all night. I didn't remember anything I'd dreamt, but it really didn't matter. What I did remember upon waking up was the music. All night, throughout each dream, I heard the same guitar riff over and over. The riff was familiar, but I did not know the name of the song or any of the words.

All I knew was that it was an Eric Clapton song with the word "gypsy" in it. Beyond that, I only recognized the tune that played incessantly in my head throughout the night. That morning I started Googling Clapton songs with the word "gypsy" in them. Turns out there are several. As I'd come across a title, I'd look it up on Spotify and play it to see if it contained the guitar portion that I had been hearing. After a few tries, I found it. The song is called "The Core" and was released in 1977, when I was three years old. I have a good memory, and I have no recollection of hearing the song anytime in the past 40 years. I looked up the lyrics and read them four times over, trying to wrap my head around what I was seeing. Here is the verse that was playing in my dream:

You can trust me; we can laugh. Together we can share our sorrow.
I will give you secrets too, an attitude that you may borrow.
Gypsy woman said to me, "One thing you must bear in your mind:
You are young and you are free, but damned if you're deceased in your
own lifetime."
Oh, you have a flame; feel it in your heart.
And down at the core is the hottest part.
We can burn without fuel.
It is burning.
It is burning.

February 14, 2019 (Valentine's Day)

I got in my car to head to work, eager as I always was to hear what songs L would sing to me to start my day. I reversed out of my garage and reached for the buttons on the dashboard to start surfing radio stations. My finger hovered over the button, on the verge of pushing it, when a mystical voice came through the speakers, singing *I've been having dreams...* I stopped my car on the driveway, my finger still lingering there, captivated by this song I had never heard before, drawn in further by each word. I put my car in park, closed my eyes, and allowed myself three minutes to just float. The song was "Trampoline" by Shaed.

I've been having dreams
Splashin' in a summer stream
Trip and I fall in
I wanted it to happen
My body turns to ice
Crushin' weight of paradise
Solid block of gold
Lying in the cold
I feel right at home
Wait if I'm on fire
How am I so deep in love?
When I dream of dying I never feel so loved

February 23, 2019

I stepped out onto the balcony of my hotel on a crisp but sunny morning in Southern California, where I was visiting a dear friend. I breathed in the fresh air and looked down at the palm of my hand. A rainbow sat squarely in the center. L was literally holding my hand. Two more then appeared, radiant and distinct, on the top of each foot. Clearly, L was ready to join me for my morning walk.

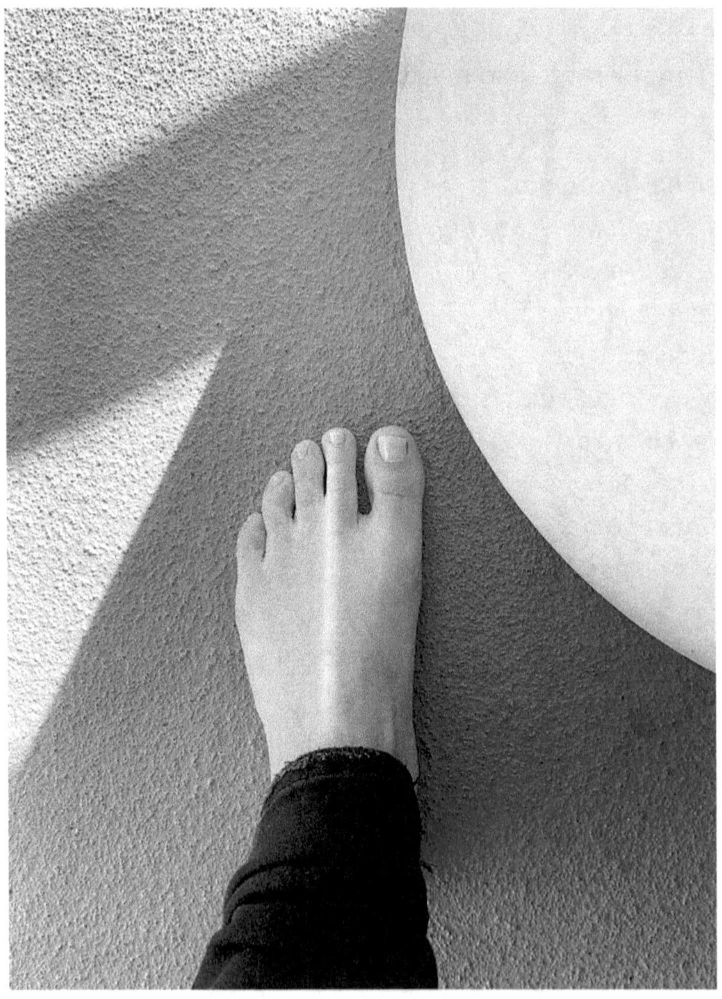

February 23, 2019.

March 7, 2019

Once again music permeated my dreams throughout the night. Only, this time

I recognized the song that was playing on repeat. It was Bette Midler's "The Rose." It came out in 1979, when I was five years old. At the time, my sister and I loved it, and we memorized every word. I had not heard it in 40 years, but the lyrics came back to me immediately, the last line singing in my head as I awoke.

Just remember in the winter,
Far beneath the bitter snow,
Lies the seed that, with the sun's love, in the spring becomes the rose.

March 14, 2019

Lisa and I had become good friends, and she texted me to let me know that it was the 35th anniversary of her mom Julie's passing, and that she was certain Julie and L were together, guiding her in her daily work. We wondered aloud when and how the rainbow would show up. It wasn't a question of if it would; it was simply a question of when and in what form.

I wanted to go for a run that evening, but it was pouring rain, so while Jaz was at dance class I went to the gym and hopped on a treadmill. The small TV monitor that was attached to the machine was airing the iHeartRadio Music Awards. I usually turn the TVs off when I'm working out, preferring to listen to my own playlist, but I spontaneously decided to watch and listen to the award show while I ran. About five minutes in, the announcer introduced the next performer. "Please welcome Kacey Musgraves singing her new solo 'Rainbow.'" I texted Lisa as fast as I could.

Me: If you're near a TV turn on the iHeartMusic Awards

Lisa: Literally watching right now, was about to text you!

Together, Lisa from her couch and I from the treadmill, we listened to a beautiful, tear-jerking live performance. Despite the millions of people who were watching, it felt like we were the only two people in the world being serenaded by our beloved Julie and L.

Oh tie up your bow, take off your coat and take a look around
Everything is alright now
'Cause the sky is finally open, the rain and wind stopped blowin'
But you're stuck out in that same old storm again
Let go of your umbrella
Cuz darlin' I'm just tryin' to tell ya that there's always been a rainbow
hangin' over your head

Lisa: *Whoa! We got our rainbow!* Me: *There they are!*

March 16, 2019

Jaz and I were shopping for a birthday present for my mom at our favorite little gift shop. While I was busy looking at scented candles and lotions for my mom, Jaz was browsing the jewelry.

"Mom, come look at this," she called me to where she was. There was a display of rainbow necklaces and earrings. Together, we both said we should get a necklace for Lisa—it seemed fitting. We picked out a simple necklace with a small horizontal bar of gems in traditional rainbow colors. As the shop owner was carefully wrapping it and curling ribbons to decorate the box, I became acutely aware of the music playing in the background of the store.

"Jaz, listen to this." Bette Midler began singing "The Rose."

March 19, 2019

Harrison and I were having lunch at the Metropolitan Club of the Sears Tower (officially, it's now the Willis Tower, but it will always be Sears to me). I had met Harrison through a mutual connection, and although he was at least 15 years my junior, he had become an important part of my support system. He had taken a keen interest in the still-unresolved legal case over the sexual abuse in the summer of 2013, and he was leaving no stone unturned in trying to get justice. Though he had not known L in life, through researching the case, reading her poetry, and listening to me talk about her, he had come to have a deep bond with her, and he felt compelled to help in any way he could. I had told him I was working on writing her story, and it turned out he was a writer himself, with knowledge and connections about the world of publishing. He offered to help in any way he could, and he read an initial draft of Part I of the manuscript.

"How are you going to end the story?" he asked.

"I'm not sure yet. But I'll know it when I see it. L will help me."

"Yeah, that sounds right."

March 20, 2019

I had been feeling off-center for about a week, and I wasn't sure why. I glanced at my phone and noticed the date, and it quickly made sense. It was the first day of spring. I had learned over the eight months since L's passing that the changing of seasons was hard for me. Even if I wasn't consciously thinking about it, my body knew. I would be thrown into a physical state of disequilibrium and would have to recalibrate my center and sense of balance with each new end and each new beginning.

My sister texted me that evening.

Are you someplace with clear skies? The moonrise tonight will be gorgeous. Around 8:00.

I got in my car just after 8:00. "The Chain" was just coming on the radio (97.1 to be exact). "Of course," I said out loud. "Of course." I drove the mile and a half to the beach with my stereo blasting. When I got there, I felt the same gravitational force that pulled me to the shore in September, and once again, I ran to the water's edge with an almost frenetic desperation. The full moon was burnt orange; a massive pumpkin in the black sky. It hung, a breath above the horizon, casting a long, golden shadow over the lake. It was the second time I had stood there immobile and breathless as I watched the moon rise over the lake, wrapped in L's unquestionable energy.

I stayed for a long time, watching the moon slowly climb in the sky, as L led me from winter into spring.

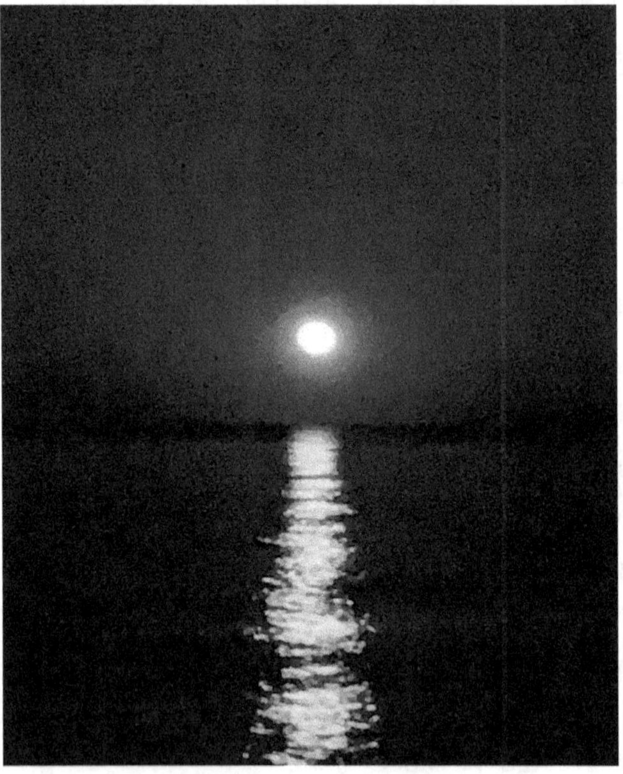

Moonrise over Lake Michigan, March 20, 2019.

EPILOGUE

Over the past several months, Lisa has become one of my most cherished friends. When we are together, L will inevitably pop in to say hi. Lisa will take on L's mannerisms, her tone of voice, her vernacular, and her sense of comedic timing. She will call or text me periodically when L has a specific message to relay, and she always delivers it with perfect accuracy and in L's own uniquely distinctive words. Independent of me, Lisa has developed a relationship with L in her own right. Although she never knew L in life, she has come to know her now, and they have created their own bond. She tells me that L is helping her in her own work, and we are both astounded that L's personality and spirit are so fully intact.

For a long time, during the course of L's illness and in the days following her death, I felt that I had failed at the singular thing I was meant to do in this lifetime. As parents, we want to be able to heal our children and take away their pain. The one thing I wanted most to do I couldn't, and I felt I had let L down profoundly. But L would not let me stay in that place for long. Her mission in death has been no different than her mission in life; her quest to bring truth to the world is uncompromised by her transition. Through her passing, she has helped me realize my truth, or at least a part of it. I can't claim to have it all figured out—she teaches me something new every day— but here is what I know at the moment: I know, beyond a shadow of a doubt, that L has not gone anywhere; she is right here by my side. And I know, because L has shown me, that it was never actually my job to heal her physical body—nobody could have done that. It was my job to nurture her soul, to help her find her way home, and to be a conduit for her soul's work.

The truth that L has taught me is that our life's work does not end when our hearts stop beating. Our ability to make a difference and to fulfill our soul's purpose does not reside within flesh and bone; it lives within our spirit and divinely guides the people we love, who then carry it even further. I have learned that relationships with the people we love don't need to end when they die—that is a choice we can make. We can choose to have only memories, or we can choose to keep these relationships active, alive, and growing, soul to soul.

L has never wavered from her purpose. She was and is a seeker and teacher of truth. I was not thinking about it in that way when I first opened my computer and began writing. I was simply trying to get her story told, to capture her essence, to honor and pay tribute to this exceptional girl I was lucky enough to call mine, and to tell her how much I love her. In the process of doing this, I've uncovered my own truth. And I realize now *that is why* L demanded I write it. That was her plan all along. She guided me every step of the way, and she knew exactly what she was doing. She held my hand through each word, cheering me on enthusiastically as I came closer and closer to figuring it out, "You got this, Mom, keep going; you're almost there!" culminating in my ultimate revelation that her job was to tell her truth so that others, including myself, could discover theirs. That is her gift to us all. That is her lasting impact. My hope is that in sharing her truth in these pages I have helped her fulfill that promise.

No sooner than I'd typed what I thought was my last word, did L draw me back one more time. I had written that last sentence above, smiled knowingly up at L, closed my computer, and gone to join Jaz on the couch on a lazy Sunday morning. She was watching SpongeBob, and two of L's favorite episodes came on. First was "Big Pink Loser," where Patrick tries to take the lid off a jar and SpongeBob says his classic, oft-quoted (in our household) line "The lid, the lid, the lid, the lid, the lid, lid, lid, lid, lid, lid." Following a commercial break for sour spray candy and inflatable cows, we saw "Best Day Ever," which featured... wait for it... L's all-time favorite song, entitled, you guessed it, "Best Day Ever." Together, Jaz, L, and I sang along with SpongeBob at the top of our lungs... "It's the best day ever!"

That's how she told me the story was complete. That's how I knew we got it right.

In the time since L passed, I have had days where my body has ached so deeply to hold her that I couldn't breathe. And I have had days when I've felt that L was more alive and vibrant now than when she was actually living; her spirit now freed from layers of pain and unencumbered by a body that turned on her.

I have found dozens of singular dimes, seen scores of ravens fly overhead, watched the sun peek out from the clouds during thunderstorms, and heard songs old and new, whose lyrics seemed to be written for L, or perhaps even by L. I have found surprising sanctuary in the Soul Cycle studio where I have danced with L to *Glee*'s version of "Raise Your Glass," laughed to "Another One Bites the Dust" and The Back Street Boys (*"Milk your udders, moo moo"*), where I have sung out loud to "Dream On," "Don't Stop Believin'," "Free Fallin'," and "Running Down a Dream," where I have cried to Pink's

"I am Here," Mumford and Sons' "Guiding Light" and "Beloved," and Kacey Musgrave's "Rainbow." I have seen hundreds of rainbows—in the sky, during snowstorms, in water glasses, in my car, on walls and floors and ceilings and chairs and balconies and showers and countertops and refrigerators. They have held my hand, danced on my toes, sat in my lap, and kissed my lips.

As I was writing this story, several people asked me if there was going to be an overarching message, or what I wanted people to take from it. I have struggled to answer these questions. I don't think there is one message, or one takeaway. Like L, the story is multifaceted and complex. It is a story of exceptionality and agony, courage and grit. It is a story of brilliance and prescience and wit. It is a story of anguish and hope, acceptance and spirituality.

It is a story of knowing who you are and knowing your innermost truth. It is a story that I hope raises awareness about invisible pain, inspires medical research, gives voice to those who have been abused, ignites a desire to fight for social justice and equality, and shows just how able disabled people can be. It is a story that I hope provides some modicum of comfort for those who are grieving; grieving for loved ones suffering on earth and grieving for those who have passed. It is a story of the triumph of the spirit despite the failure of the body.

It is a story that challenges our ideas of what it means to live and what it means to die. It is a story of grief and of finding salvation in some of the most unexpected ways and of giving yourself permission to find it. It is a story of truth and determination and liberation. It is a story of knowing that whatever your faith or background, there are certain bonds that can never be broken.

And, most importantly, it is a story of love.

ACKNOWLEDGEMENTS

There are so many people who have supported me and Jaz and L. It is hard to know where to begin. Thank you to L's medical team, Dr. Lubenow, Dr. Gary, Nan, Robin, Melissa, Sharon, Jessica; her amazing friends who brought her so much joy, Agatha, Bill, Pashi, Wes, Amara, Ashton, Madison, Ms. K; the friends and support system who wrapped their arms around me and Jaz and never let go, Marcy, Linda, Julie, Donna, Cristina, Robyn; Amy, who showed up at the bottom of my stairs and has bravely and boldly channeled L to tell me the things I needed to hear; she has never steered me wrong; Harrison, who selflessly jumped in to help me get L's story told; Melanie, who helped me get L's message out to the world; Jen, who gave Lisa the rainbow necklace that found its way to me and who edited this manuscript with love and compassion; Mia, who loves L and Jaz as if they were her own and who takes care of all of us every day; S, my gentle, quiet rock; my family who quite literally would do anything for me, Jaz and L at any moment, Mom, Dad, Brigitte, and D; Lisa Nitzkin, who showed me that angels really do exist right here on earth and who has given me a gift I can never possibly repay; my Jaz, who has the biggest heart of anyone I have ever known, who heals me every day with the "Jazzy love," who has shown incredible courage, grace, and compassion, who sees goodness and beauty in the world around her, and who inspires me in ways I cannot express.

I love you Jazzy. And, of course, L, who blessed me with 15 years in this world and a lifetime in my heart and soul. Thank you for helping me find my truth, for telling me exactly how you would show up, and for doing it so flawlessly. I will forever be in awe of you. I can't wait to see what you show me next. I love you baby girl, always.

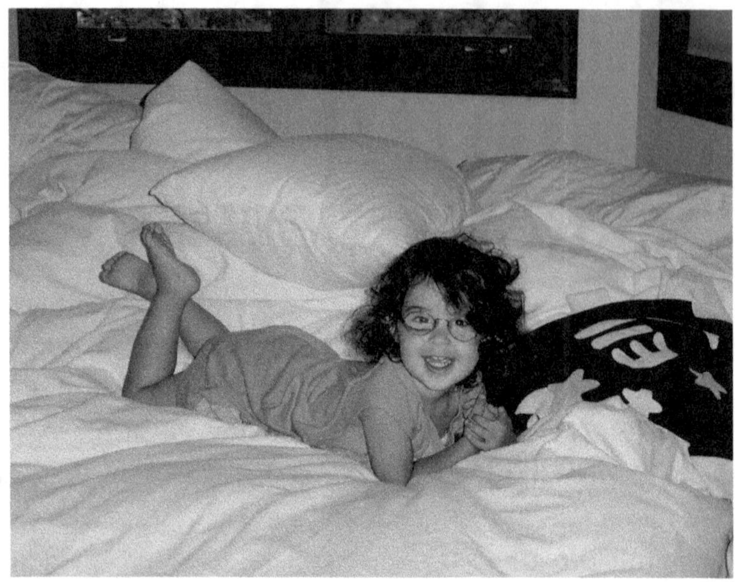

My girl

Thank you for taking the time to read our book.

If you would like to leave us an honest review, please visit our book page on Amazon: https://www.amazon.com/dp/Bo8BZYWLCQ.

RESOURCES

Not your inspiration (L Grey's podcast; 14 episodes total)
https://www.youtube.com/watch?v=7ZG-f8iOU6o

Burning Limb Foundation
www.burninglimb.com

Human Rights Campaign
www.hrc.org

True Colors Fund
www.truecolorsunited.org

The Trevor Project
www.thetrevorproject.org

National Suicide Prevention Lifeline
https://suicidepreventionlifeline.org/

SONGS

Free
Producer: Steve Lillywhite, Phish

Time to Say Goodbye
Label: East West
Songwriters: Francesco Sartori, Lucio Quarantotto
Producer: Frank Peterson

Dream On
Label: Columbia
Songwriter: Steven Tyler
Producer: Adrian Barber

Everybody
Label: Jive
Songwriters: Denniz Pop, Max Martin
Producers: Denniz Pop, Max Martin

Don't Stop Believin'
Label: Columbia
Songwriters: Steve Perry, Jonathan Cain, Neal Schon
Producers: Kevin Elson, Mike Stone

Another One Bites the Dust
Label: EMI, Elektra
Songwriter: John Deacon
Producers: Queen, Mack

The Chain
Label: Warner Bros.
Songwriters: Lindsey Buckingham, Mick Fleetwood, Christine McVie, John McVie, Stevie Nicks
Producers: Fleetwood Mac, Ken Caillat, Richard Dashut

The Waiting
Label: Backstreet
Songwriter: Tom Petty
Producers: Tom Petty, Jimmy Iovine

Free Fallin'
Label: MCA
Songwriters: Tom Petty, Jeff Lynne
Producers: Tom Petty, Jeff Lynne, Mike Campbell

The Core
Label: RSO
Songwriters: Eric Clapton, Marcy Levy
Producer: Glyn Johns

Trampoline
Label: Photo Finish
Songwriters: Chelsea Lee, Max Ernst, Spencer Ernst
Producers: Alex Mendoza, Grant Eadie, Shaed

Rainbow
Label: MCA Nashville
Songwriters: Kacey Musgraves, Natalie Hemby, Shane McAnally
Producers: Ian Fitchuk, Daniel Tashian, Kacey Musgraves

The Rose
Label: Atlantic
Songwriter: Amanda McBroom
Producer: Paul A. Rothchild

Best Day Ever
Songwriters: Andy Paley, Tom Kenny

ABOUT THE AUTHORS

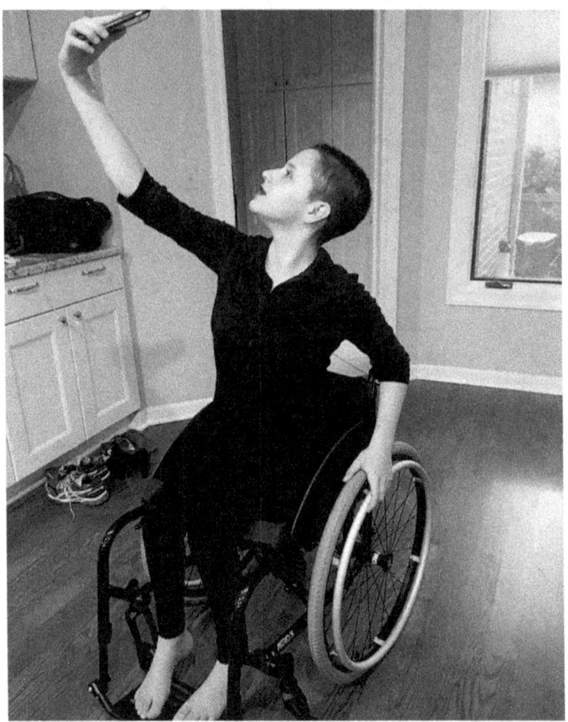

L Grey - L, who's at the center of the book, was determined to tell her own story. Precocious, courageous, and inspirational, L was wise beyond her years. She wrote with furious conviction about being misunderstood and seldom believed, being wheelchair-bound and then bed-ridden, and about dealing with constant, torturous physical pain. Nevertheless, L's writing shows pure resiliency in its empathy, strength and forgiveness.

Podcast: Not your inspiration
https://www.youtube.com/watch?v=7ZG-f8iOU6o

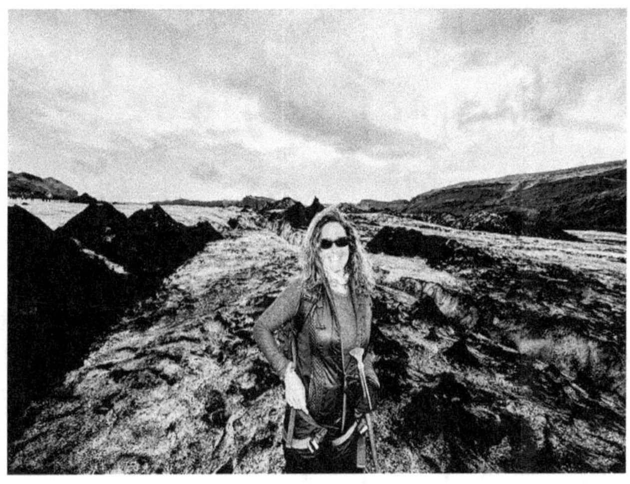

Vanessa Lynn, Ph.D. - Vanessa never set out to be an author, but L had other plans for her. She is a mother first, and then a consultant. She holds a bachelor's degree in psychology from the University of Pennsylvania, a master's degree in counseling psychology from Northwestern University, and a Ph.D. in organization behavior from the Kellogg School of Management. She is the proud mother of her two beautiful daughters, L and Jaz. She currently lives in the Chicago area with Jaz and their dog, Evie.

Visit: www.ravensandrainbows.com

email: RavensRainbows1112@gmail.com

Facebook:
https://www.facebook.com/Ravens-Rainbows-103644218062675

Instagram: https://www.instagram.com/ravensandrainbows1112/

About Defining Moments Press

Built for aspiring authors who are looking to share transformative ideas with others throughout the world, Defining Moments Press offers life coaches, healers, business professionals, and other non-fiction or self-help authors a comprehensive solution to get their book published without taking years or investing their life savings.

Defining Moments Press prides itself on bringing readers and authors together to find tools and solutions for everyday challenges from people who have overcome them.

As an alternative to self-publishing or signing with a major publishing house - we offer full profits to our authors, low-priced author copies, and simple contract terms.

Most authors get stuck trying to navigate the technical end of publishing. The comprehensive publishing services offered by Defining Moments Press mean that your book will be designed by an experienced graphic artist, available in printed, hard copy format, and coded for all eBook readers, including Kindle, iPad, Nook, and more.

We handle all of the technical aspects of your book creation so you can spend more time focusing on your business that makes a difference for other people.

Defining Moments Press founder, publisher and #1 bestselling author, Melanie Warner, has over 20 years of experience as a writer, publisher, master life coach and accomplished entrepreneur.

You can learn more about Warner's innovative approach to self-publishing or take advantage of free trainings and education at: www.MyDefiningMoments.com or email us:
melanie@MyDefiningMoments.com

Defining Moments Book Publishing

If you're like many authors, you have wanted to write a book for a long time, maybe you have even started a book... but somehow, as hard as you have tried to make your book a priority - other things keep getting in the way.

Some authors have fears about their ability to write or whether or not anyone will value what they write or buy their book. For others, the challenge is making the time to write their book or having accountability to finish it.

It's not just finding the time and confidence to write that is an obstacle. Most authors get overwhelmed with the logistics of finding an editor, finding a support team, hiring an experienced designer, and figuring out all the technicalities of writing, publishing, marketing and launching a book. Others have actually written a book and might have even published it but did not find a way to make it profitable.

For more information on how to participate in our next Defining Moments Author Training program visit: www.MyDefiningMoments.com. Or you can email melanie@MyDefiningMoments.com

OTHER BOOKS BY DEFINING MOMENTS PRESS

Defining Moments: Coping With the Loss of a Child - by Melanie Warner

Defining Moments SOS: Stories of Survival - by Melanie Warner and Amber Torres

Write your Bestselling Book in 8 Weeks or Less and Make a Profit - Even if No One Has Ever Heard of You - by Melanie Warner

Beyond Brilliant: Roadmap From Fear to Courage – by Shiran Cohen

Rise, Fight, Love, Repeat: Ignite Your Morning Fire – by Jeff Wickersham

Life Mapping: Decoding the Blueprint of Your Soul - by Karen Loenser

www.ingramcontent.com/pod-product-compliance
Lightning Source LLC
Chambersburg PA
CBHW071210240726
48654CB00009B/722